Health Yourself

Health Yourself

The Candy, Booze & Sex Prescription!

by KEN DAVIS, MD

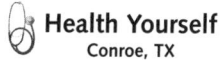

Health Yourself
Conroe, TX

Copyright © 2003 Ken Davis

All rights reserved. No part of this book may be reproduced or transmitted in any form or by any means, electronic or mechanical, including photocopying, recording, or by any information storage and retrieval system, without permission in writing from the publisher.

Published by Health Yourself
508 Medical Center Blvd.
Conroe, TX 77304

Publisher's Cataloging-in-Publication Data
Davis, Ken
    Health yourself : the candy, booze, and sex prescription / Ken Davis.--Conroe, Tex. : Health Yourself, 2003.

    p. ; cm.
    ISBN: 0-9726434-0-0

    1. Health behavior. 2. Health attitudes. 3. Health.

RA776.9 .D38 2003   2002115383
613-dc21   0303

Book coordination by Jenkins Group, Inc. • www.bookpublishing.com
Cover design by Leslie Tane
Cover illustrated by Nancy Parsons
Interior design by Theresa Baehr
Printed in the United States of America

07 06 05 04 03 • 5 4 3 2 1

Acknowledgments and Dedication

This book is dedicated to my mother, Nona Davis, and to the memory of my father, Bob L. Davis. Their support and sacrifices made me and these efforts possible.

The seemingly interminable gestation period of this book would have been overwhelmingly unbearable without the support and indulgence of my wife Kitty. Her wise counsel and willingness to ply her needlecraft during my prolonged sessions at the keyboard maintained our respective sanity and preserved the 32-year investment we have made in our marriage.

The "other women" in my life, my office nurse (and cousin) Debbie along with my receptionist Rachel, are due credit for enduring my surreptitious retreats to the keyboard during office hours. My forays into the literary pursuit often disrupted the schedule, thwarted their daily routines, and virtually assured there would be no structure or predictability in the flow of the day's activities.

Our daughters Hilary and Ashley also contributed to the effort significantly and provided encouragement and inspiration.

I would not have had the insight or courage to undertake this project without the stimulus provided by my colleagues in the

Health Yourself

National Speakers Association, who often repeated the mantra "If you have a speech, you've got a book, too."

My thanks to Dr. Dale Anderson and Dr. Jo Lichten, who reviewed the manuscript and made a number of excellent suggestions and provided the testimonial quotes.

Leah Nicholson, Kelli Leader, Rebecca Chown, and the staff at The Jenkins Group were of invaluable assistance in the editing, composition, and design of the book. My good friend and graphic design artist Nancy Parsons captured the spirit and essence of my message in her artwork that graces the cover.

To put the literary gestation in perspective, during the time I spent on this book we have changed presidents, endured a terrorist attack, fought a war, and Kitty and I will have experienced our first two grandchildren.

Contents

Introduction
ix

Section One
Pantry Prevention
1

Section Two
Pleasurable Pursuits
65

Section Three
Positive Passions
99

Introduction

The inferior doctor treats actual illness;
the average doctor treats impending illness;
the superior doctor prevents illness.

Ancient Chinese Proverb

How many times have you been to the doctor and received advice about giving up, cutting out, or eliminating enjoyable behaviors and activities? Most of my physician colleagues and I are very adept at dispensing this type of advice, but we have no training in how to make positive recommendations, especially ones that might result in adding pleasure or enjoyment to a patient's life. Over my 25 years of practice, I have found myself asking the same question over and over: how can I prescribe something fun and pleasurable to help people live longer and happier lives instead of dispensing those negative prescriptions?

Finally, I decided to find a new and better approach after one of my patients, Leroy Farkus, opened my eyes by telling me, "Doc, I've read so much about the negative effects of eating and drinking that I decided to give up reading." Leroy, a 67-year-old retired logger, had just experienced his third heart attack in five years. As he was leaving the hospital I recited the usual medical litany of "thou-shalt-nots" that had obviously failed him again. Leroy rolled his eyes,

Health Yourself

shook his head, and said, "Doc, if you ask me to cut out anything else, there won't be anything left to cut out except paper dolls."

I resolved then and there to come up with an approach that would allow patients to make better and more informed choices regarding their health. I also resolved that most of those choices would be positive and enjoyable ones. "Stop smoking and stop using tobacco" was the only negative advice I chose to retain from my list of negatives. I did away with advice like "Lose weight," "Stop drinking," and "Cut out sweets." As I began to search the medical literature and popular press, I noticed articles coinciding with my philosophy of adding to rather than subtracting from patients' lives as I treated them for their medical problems. Many of these articles also promoted the idea that patients can be more directly involved in their health care decisions, a notion that I also wanted to incorporate into my practice.

I collected and studied those articles for several years and molded them into a television program, *Health Yourself: Prevention from A to Z*, that appeared on the Health Sciences Television Network. Patients as well as doctors and other members of the health care team embraced the concepts and I began to get requests to make presentations explaining the "Candy, Booze, and Sex Prescription." At these programs people began to request a copy of the book, and I would sheepishly explain that I did not yet have a book on the subject. After several such requests, I made another resolution: to put the information in book form and to enlist as many patients as possible to spread the word of my novel approach to medical care.

All those old cowboy movies I'd watched as a child finally paid off when I came up with the idea of "deputizing." In the days of the Old West, a sheriff could take civilians off the street and make them law enforcement officers by deputizing them in a time of crisis or special need.

Today we are facing such a time. We Americans are killing ourselves as the result of our poor lifestyle choices. The effect is painfully evident when you examine Table 1, which outlines the top 15 causes of death in America today.

Introduction

The 15 leading causes of death in the general poplution, 1997

Rank*	Cause of death†	Percent of total deaths	Death rate**	1997***	Percent change, 1996-1997***	Percent change, 1979-1997***	Ratio, male to female***	Ratio, black to white***
NA	All causes	100.0	864.7	479.1	-2.5	-17.0	1.6	1.5
1	Diseases of the heart	31.4	271.6	130.5	-3.0	-34.6	1.8	1.5
2	Malignant neoplasms, including neoplasms of lymphatic and hematopoietic tissues	23.3	210.6	125.6	-1.8	-4.0	1.4	1.3
3	Cerebrovascular diseases	6.9	59.7	25.9-1.9	-37.7	1.2	1.8	
4	COPDs and allied conditions	4.7	40.7	21.1	0.5	44.5	1.5	0.8
5	Accidents and adverse effects	4.1	35.7	30.1	-1.0	-29.8	2.4	1.2
	Motor vehicle accidents	1.9	16.2	15.9	-1.0	-31.5	2.1	1.1
	All other accidents and adverse effects	2.2	19.5	14.2	0.0	-27.6	2.8	1.4
6	Pneumonia and influenza	3.7	32.3	12.9	0.8	15.2`1.5	1.4	
7	Diabetes melitus	2.7	23.4	13.5	-0.7	37.8	1.2	2.4
8	Suicide	1.3	11.4	10.6	-1.9	-9.4	4.2	0.6
9	Nephritis, nephrotic syndrome, and nephrosis	1.1	9.5	4.4	2.3	2.3	1.5	2.6
10	Chronic liver disease and cirrhosis	1.1	9.4	7.4	-1.3	-38.3	2.3	1.2
11	Alzheimer's disease	1.0	8.4	4.2	0.0	1250.	0.9	0.7
12	Septicemia	1.0	8.4	4.2	2.4	82.6	1.2	2.8
13	Homicide and legal intervention	0.9	7.4	8.0	-5.9	-21.6	3.8	6.0
14	HIV infection	0.7	6.2	5.8	47.7	Data lacking	3.5	7.5
15	Atherosclerosis	0.7	6.0	2.1	-4.5	-63.2	1.3	1.0
NA	All other causes	153.4	132.9	NA	NA	NA	NA	NA

Key: COPDs, chronic obstructive pulmonary diseases; NA, not applicable.
* Based on number of deaths
† Based on the *Ninth Revision international Classification of Diseases,* 1975
** Per 100,000 population
*** Age-adjusted death rates per 100,000 US standard population

Source: Hoyert DL, Kochanek KD, Murphy SL. Deaths: final data for 1997, *National Vital Statistics Reports.* Hyattsville, Md: National Center for Health Statistics; June 30, 1999, DHHS publication (PHS) 99-1120. Available at http://www.cdc.gov/nchswww/releases/99facts/99sheets/97mortal.htm. Accessed August 2, 1999

Each year we have over 300,000 premature deaths from obesity (mostly because it causes diabetes) and more than 450,000 Americans die from smoking-related illnesses. Doctors are powerless to make a significant

Health Yourself

impact on these numbers without enlisting the help and participation of their patients.

Like the old time sheriff, I will deputize you to become a "doctor." You won't have a diploma to adorn your wall or a shingle to hang out, but you will be a doctor in the original Greek meaning of the word that translates as "teacher." By using the information in this book, you can teach yourself, your family members, and your loved ones to make better and wiser choices that will help prevent you and them from becoming one of the statistics mentioned above. We will go one step beyond the Chinese proverb's definition of a superior doctor and make each of you an *ultimate* "doctor" as you learn to practice the art of PRO-vention, one of the original concepts on which this book is based.

PRO-vention focuses on adding positive aspects to your life that are enjoyable as well as beneficial for your health. *Prevention*, a term most of us are familiar with, means trying to keep something negative from happening. The goal of PRO-vention, on the other hand, is to make something positive happen. Practicing "prevention" means getting childhood immunizations and, for adults, getting your flu shot so you won't come down with a case of the "killer" flu. Pap smears, mammograms, and blood tests for prostate cancer are early-warning systems of prevention designed to detect disease in time to allow a cure. These measures are necessary and beneficial, but they are sometimes expensive and seldom enjoyable.

The second original concept in this book is a new definition of health. The dictionary defines health as a noun or a thing one has. "PRO-vention" is based on the new concept that health is a verb, an action word, something you *do* rather than something you *have*. Looking at the concept of health from this new angle will give you a better idea of what it means to "health yourself." Health, however, is not the ultimate goal of our efforts to improve our lives. I once heard someone jokingly say, "Health is just the slowest rate at which you can die." The goal of PRO-vention is not to prolong the dying process but to accelerate the living process so you can fulfill the Old Testament concept of "shalom." This ancient but timeless ideal

Introduction

refers to living in a way that brings together the fullness of life in the physical, mental, and spiritual realms.

Of course, you will still need your fully licensed physician for certain preventive measures and procedures. See the list below for the most effective routine preventive measures.

10 most effective preventive services

(Adapted from a 1999 issue of *Family Practice News* reported in *American Family Physician*)

- Childhood immunizations
- Flu vaccine for people over 65
- Pneumonia vaccine for people over 65
- Tobacco use screening and smoking cessation advice for people over 18
- Blood pressure screening
- Hormone replacement therapy for women at or near menopause
- Folic acid intake for women of childbearing age
- Newborn screening
- Screening for cervical cancer (pap smears)
- Cholesterol screening

In this book I will show you not only how to take responsibility for your own health, but how to enjoy yourself thoroughly along the way. PRO-vention has three components, each of which is addressed in separate sections of the book. "P" stands for Pantry Prevention, which deals with what we eat and drink. In this section you learn that enjoying positive and pleasurable things such as candy and alcohol can also yield health benefits.

"R" is for recreation or enjoyable activities as outlined in the Pleasurable Pursuits section, which teaches you the health benefits of physical activity, an active sex life, and other enjoyable pastimes.

Health Yourself

"O" comes from "emotion," or the attitudinal and spiritual aspects of our lives. In Section III, Positive Passions, you will learn the value of positive relationships, religion, humor, and service to others.

Practicing the principles of PRO-vention means adding activities to your life that are both beneficial and enjoyable. Most everyone enjoys eating, drinking, and making love and I heartily endorse the combination of all three and actually prescribe them as a way to achieve a longer and healthier life. Once you become your own "doctor" of PRO-vention, you can write a "Candy, Booze, and Sex" PRO-scription for yourself.

But first, consider this: in the early 1900s, the average life expectancy was 47 years for a man and slightly longer for a woman. Today, experts set our life expectancy at about 74 years for men and about 79 years for women. Those born in the recent past should live even longer. Other experts tell us that the human body is designed to last well past the age of 90 years, and one researcher even claims that anyone who dies before they reach the age of 100 has died prematurely. The Bible says, "He who dies at a hundred will be thought a mere youth…" (Isaiah 65:20). Our overall health and length of life are due to factors such as access to medical care, our physical environment, social circumstances, our genetic make up, and our behavioral choices, arguably the most important of the five factors.

While our health is determined by a complex interplay among these five factors, medical experts agree that nearly three-fourths of all illnesses and diseases are directly related to our poor lifestyle choices. An article in *Time* magazine (February 5, 2001) confirmed the assertion by noting that "Doctors believe that as much as 70% of all chronic diseases in the U.S. – from diabetes and high blood pressure to heart disease and even some cancers – can be warded off with some timely, sensible changes in lifestyle."

Thus, the behavioral choices we make in the areas of diet, activity, and emotion or attitude can have either a positive or negative impact on our health. One group of researchers found diet and activity accounted for 14% of premature deaths, just behind smoking and tobacco use, the grand prizewinners that account for nearly 20% of all deaths.

Introduction

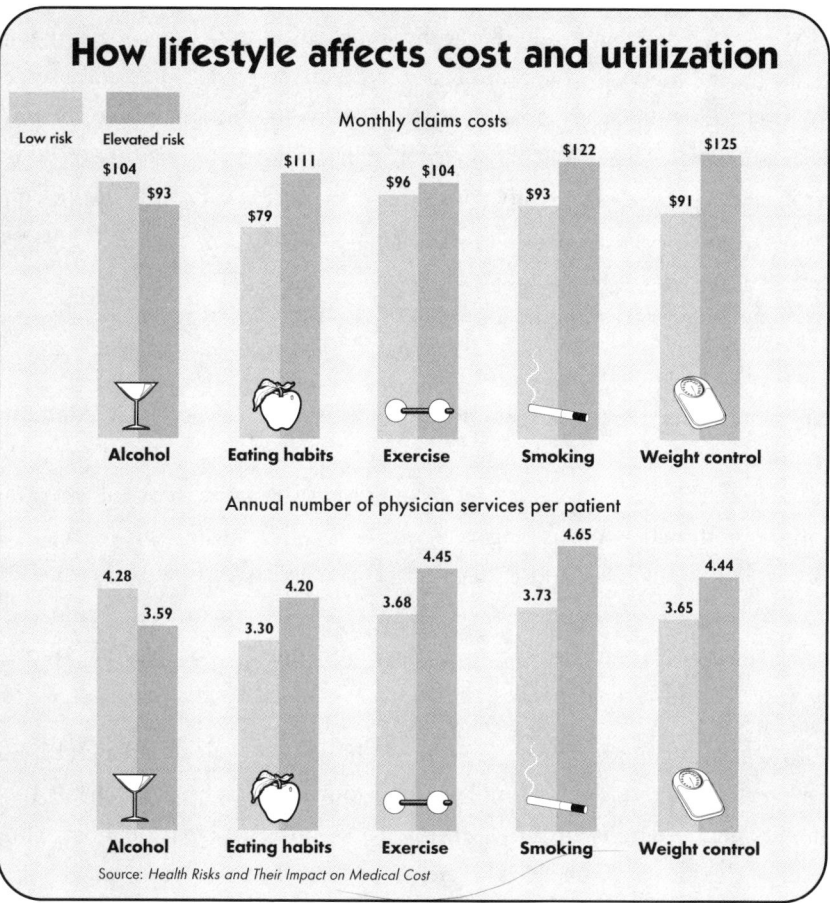

Source: Health Risks and Their Impact on Medical Cost

Will changing your choices toward healthier options pay off? According to one medical researcher, the answer is a resounding yes! Dr. Thomas Perls, the lead investigator in the study of health habits of those who have lived to 100 years of age, tells us, "Those who take appropriate health measures can add as many as 10 quality years to their lives – and those who don't can subtract a decade." The chart above shows the higher health care costs associated with various behavioral choices. Whenever I hear comments about the high cost of medical care, I am reminded that "health care" is relatively inexpensive. It's "sick care," the price of our poor choices, that accounts for escalating medical expenses. Incorporating the recommendations in this book is much less expensive than paying for the consequences of our less than perfect decisions.

Health Yourself

However, please keep in mind that the information in this book is intended as general medical advice and is not to be interpreted as personal advice for each individual. My goal is to stimulate your thought processes and increase your interest in taking responsibility for certain aspects of your own health. Always talk with your doctor or health care provider before making any changes in your approach to your healthcare or before incorporating any of the ideas and recommendations you read in this book into your personal plan of medical care.

Please also keep in mind that of these five influential factors, the only one we cannot change is our genetics or heredity. We cannot pick different ancestors, but in this book I will give you the information you need to make better and healthier choices in the other four areas that will also add some refreshing spice and zing to your life. We all want to "die young…as late in life as possible," and PRO-vention teaches us to how to reach that goal by focusing on the quality of life as well as the quantity. Reading and using this book as a resource can help you to achieve a longer, fuller, more productive and healthier life.

Although most of the information in this book comes from research based on credible medical sources and medical journals, I cannot vouch for the validity and reliability of those who performed the research or those who publish the results. Even reliable scientific medical information can change as quickly as the Texas weather. Visiting www.healthyourselves.com is another easy way to keep abreast of the latest information on PRO-vention, and the following story illustrates the need for constantly updating our information and knowledge in the areas involving our health and wellness.

The Parable of *Yo La Tengo*

One of my favorite baseball stories demonstrates that what happens in baseball has a wider application to life in general. When Richie Ashburn played outfield with the hapless 1961 New York Mets, he frequently collided with his teammate Elio Chacon who spoke only Spanish and did not understand what Ashburn meant when he yelled "I got it" as the two of

Introduction

them closed in on the fly ball coming their way. After several of these mishaps, Ashburn asked his manager Casey Stengel for a solution to this communication problem. Stengel thought quietly for a few moments, then answered in his inimitable style, "Richie, you need to learn three words: *'Yo la tengo.'* That means *'I've got it'* in Spanish."

Ashburn practiced the phrase for days and then during a real game, he and Chacon were closing in on the fly ball and Ashburn cried out "*Yo la tengo*" and Chacon stopped in his tracks. As Ashburn was about to make the play, *BLAM!* He collided with the other outfielder who had been closing in on the ball from the other direction but who had no idea what *Yo la tengo* meant.

The moral of the story is that no matter how much we learn and no matter what kind of adjustments we make in life, we can still be blindsided by the unexpected. What you discover and learn in this book may be out of date, disproved, or expanded upon and improved before the ink dries. The constantly changing landscape of medical knowledge is precisely the reason I have developed my website. On this site you will find the same arrangement of sections as in the book and I will provide you with new information, research, and articles to keep you updated on the latest advances in medical knowledge that apply to the concept of PRO-vention. I encourage you to become a regular visitor to the website. While you're there, you can sign up for the monthly electronic newsletter so you don't become a victim of the *Yo la tengo* phenomenon.

Let's get started and explore the tantalizing and healthy pleasures in Section I, Pantry Prevention, and get ourselves involved in a food fight against the major causes of death and disability.

Section One

> *There is no difference between food and medicine.*
>
> Ancient Chinese Proverb

In the decade of the 1960s a popular phrase was, "You are what you eat." We now know this statement is more accurate than we ever thought or hoped it would be. Even so, I like what one humorist said: "If we are what we eat, we should all be French fries."

According to the American Cancer Society, one-third of all cancer deaths in the United States are due to dietary factors and by following nutritional guidelines, we could reduce cancer by 30 to 40%.

Researchers have shown that dietary choices can also make an impact on cardiovascular disease (heart attacks and stroke), the other top two killers in the United States. In 1998, researchers reviewed several years' worth of medical reports and investigations and found that those individuals with the highest intake of fruits and vegetables had the lowest risk of heart disease. A report in the January 2001 *Running and Fit News* (*RFN*) showed that women who ate nine or more servings of fruits and vegetables daily had a 31% lower risk of stroke than those women who ate only two servings a day. Eating a balanced and healthy diet can also prevent other medical conditions such as diabetes, obesity, depression, and blindness.

PANTRY PREVENTION

Health Yourself

To achieve these benefits, I want you to add enjoyable foods and beverages to your daily intake rather than focus on leaving off, eliminating, or doing without. Let's begin with breakfast and work our way through the day and see how we can enjoy the pleasures of eating while we improve our health and reduce our risk of dying prematurely from the major killers.

Breakfast

Most everyone likes to eat, some of us more than others. My Uncle Doo-Dad described himself as a light eater: "When it gets light, I start eating," he often said. Research shows that many of us don't start eating when it gets light. A study from the Baylor College of Medicine conducted between 1998-2000 found that 14% of students do not eat breakfast at all, and the percentage of breakfast dropouts increases with age. By early adulthood a full 33% of us skip breakfast altogether while many of us eat a snack in the car on the way to work and another five percent indulge in a fast-food breakfast. According to a 1998 Gallup survey, 46% of people reported spending five minutes or less on a weekday breakfast. I agree with the anonymous philosopher who said, "All happiness depends upon a leisurely breakfast."

I recommend making breakfast a regular part of your life, as doing so can lower the risk of developing depression and can also help you control your weight. According to a news brief in the May 1999 *American Family Physician* (*AFP*), nutritional scientists reported that adults ages 20 to 79 who ate breakfast daily had lower levels of emotional distress and tended to feel less stressed and depressed than those who skipped breakfast altogether. When I reviewed the research on the habits of those who lived to be over 100 years old, I found that one thing they all had in common was eating a good breakfast every day. Have you heard the old expression, "Eat like a king at breakfast, like a princess at lunch, and like a pauper at dinner"? We now know that bit of advice makes good medical sense!

These centenarians did not limit themselves to fruit and tofu, either. Many of them admitted to eating bacon and eggs as their main courses at breakfast. Eating high fat and high calorie foods at breakfast is not the healthiest

Pantry Prevention

choice every day, but if you want to splurge once or twice a week, breakfast is a good time to do it since you have all day to burn it off! Weight loss experts tell us that eating breakfast increases our chances of losing weight, as we then tend to snack less before the next meal.

Runner's World (*RW*) magazine reported in October of 2001 that for almost 2,000 people over the age of 12, those who ate ready-to-eat breakfast cereals had more healthful diets and leaner bodies than those who ate breakfast foods such as eggs, French toast, bagels, or other bread products. In this same study, scientists found that even though breakfast-eaters consumed more calories per day, they wound up weighing the same or less than those who skipped breakfast. Non-breakfast eaters tended to make up for their hunger by eating higher calorie foods later in the day.

Breakfast eaters also apparently find it easier to develop other positive health habits, as they tend to be non-smokers, to drink less alcohol, and to have healthier diets than non-breakfast eaters.

Baylor College of Medicine nutrition researcher Theresa Nicklas made an extensive study of high school students in 1998 and found that students who ate breakfast performed better in school. Nicklas also found that eating cereal for breakfast proved to be convenient, nutritious, and inexpensive. Fast-food breakfasts from the popular outlets like Burger King cost $2.38 as compared to $.78 for a bowl of cereal. Even so, only 28% of consumers in a Department of Agriculture survey believed that cereal is a good value for the money and most said it was too expensive to buy without a coupon. By the same token, breakfasts from the fast-food franchises contained nearly four times as many calories and fat as cereals and were inferior to cereal in providing nutrients such as fiber, proteins, vitamins, and minerals.

The idea of eating breakfast received a divine endorsement when Jesus told his disciples, "Come and let's have breakfast" (John 21:12). What's more, when Jesus invited his disciples to breakfast, he served them fish. This example dispels the myth that you have to eat traditional breakfast foods to get the most nutritional value. How many times have you thought about

Health Yourself

that last slice of leftover pizza for breakfast the next day? Go for it! Pizza contains tomato sauce, cheese, and bread and supplies carbohydrates, fats, and proteins. An article in the fall 2002 issue of *Well Being* (*WB*) magazine reminds us that "The only poor choices are empty calorie meals that include only fats and sweets."

The same article points out that breakfast foods that contain mostly starches (carbohydrates) can lower your blood sugar quickly and may result in hunger pangs by the middle of the morning. I've found I can avoid these mid-morning sinking spells by adding protein foods to my breakfast. High protein soy patties, low-fat cheese, yogurt, milk, and peanut butter are excellent choices to help balance out the carbohydrates.

When scientists investigated the eating habits of 3,000 individuals who lost 30 pounds or more and kept the weight off for more than a year, they found that 78% of them reported eating breakfast seven days a week. Besides losing weight, the breakfast eaters had higher energy levels than the non-breakfast eaters, according to the report in the June 2002 *RW*.

Let's look at some of the common breakfast foods we can choose from to make this first meal of the day an enjoyable treat! Here are some excellent suggestions for "creative and healthy" breakfast ideas from *WB* (September 2002):

- Omelet (using egg or egg substitute) with salsa and soy cheese
- Granola with low-fat yogurt and banana slices
- Fruit salad with cottage cheese
- Poached salmon with steamed seasonal vegetables
- Smoked salmon and tomato on a bagel with low-fat cream cheese
- Peanut butter and banana sandwich on whole wheat bread
- Tuna salad with fat-free mayonnaise over a bed of baby spinach
- Steamed halibut with lemon juice over a bed of brown rice cooked with your favorite herbs
- Grilled or broiled seafood sausage with a side of sliced tomatoes and a whole wheat English muffin

Pantry Prevention

Filtering Through the Coffee Controversy

When I think of breakfast, the first thing that comes to mind is the smell of freshly brewed coffee. According to researchers in the December 2001 *Journal of Clinical Hypertension* report, I am not alone. These investigators found that 85 to 90% of persons ages 18 to 74 report drinking coffee, and 40% drink coffee or tea three or more times daily.

However, controversy has arisen lately as to whether coffee is a "good guy" or a "bad guy." I looked over the recent research and found that sipping a little Java in moderation has no ill effects on health. According to the February 2001 *UC Berkeley Wellness Letter* (*UCBWL*), "Coffee has been blamed for causing many ailments but in nearly every instance it has been declared *not guilty*." In fact, a recent study in the winter 2002 issue of *Men's Health* (*MH*) showed that men who drank two or three cups of coffee daily had a 40% lower risk of gallstones than those who did not drink coffee regularly. Java drinkers may also benefit from a reduced risk of Parkinson's disease and an enhancement of the pain-killing effects of ibuprofen. Neither decaf coffee, caffeinated teas, or sodas had a similar protective effect.

The active ingredient in coffee is caffeine, a chemical that has a stimulating effect on the brain and central nervous system. This effect accounts for the jolt and increased mental alertness many people experience when they drink coffee. Coffee also has many other active chemicals that may share some of the beneficial effects found in tea, which we will examine later on.

Previous reports linking coffee to heart disease, high blood pressure, cancer, osteoporosis, breast cysts, infertility, and birth defects have likewise proven to have no scientific basis. Another study reported in the *UCBWL* (May 1999) found that even four or more cups of coffee a day didn't increase the risk of heart attack. However, caution is in vogue for those who drink more than four cups a day: researchers measured blood pressure and stress hormone levels after drinking 500 milligrams of caffeine (the equivalent of four cups of coffee) and found they were elevated and stayed up all day.

Health Yourself

Two cups of coffee a day may even boost your memory, especially in older adults, according to an article in the journal *Psychological Science* reported in *RW* (April 2002). Researchers also found that runners can improve their endurance and performance by taking in two milligrams of caffeine per pound of body weight an hour before beginning their activity. For example, a 150-pound person would need to consume 300 milligrams of caffeine, the equivalent of two cups of brewed coffee. Consult the accompanying chart below to learn the caffeine content of popular products containing caffeine.

Caffeine content
(in milligrams)

Coffee (eight-ounce serving)

Regular	135
Instant coffee	95
Decaffeinated coffee	5

Teas

From leaf or bag	50 per eight ounces
Bottled iced tea	42 per 16 ounces
Green tea	30 per eight ounces

Sodas (per 12-ounce serving)

Mountain Dew	55
Surge	51
Diet Coke	47
Coca Cola	45
Dr. Pepper (regular or diet)	42
Pepsi	37

Over-the-counter medications

Vivarin	200
No Doz	100

Pantry Prevention

Caffeine also lowers the perception of effort and increases the body's efficiency in burning fatty acids, thus sparing the fuel (carbohydrates) stored in leg muscles.

I like to make my coffee "half and half" by using equal parts of decaffeinated and regular. Watch out for those sophisticated coffee drinks like lattes and mochas, as they are often made with whole milk that adds unwanted calories and fat grams. A 12-ounce latte made with whole milk weighs in with 200 calories and 10 grams of fat. Ask for a "skinny latte" made with non-fat milk and you can shave off a hundred calories and get only a single gram of fat.

The main negative side effect of coffee for me occurs when my wife gets upset with me for spilling coffee on my clothes or on the carpet. I was surprised to learn that my morning jolt of java may be harmful to the furniture but may not be quite so toxic to my teeth and may even help prevent cavities. Coffee contains numerous chemicals that impart its flavor and aroma and these compounds stick to your teeth, protecting them from the bacteria that cause tooth decay.

So, if you are generally healthy, you can safely enjoy three or four cups of coffee a day and get the mental boost you need to make it through the day, though you may notice that drinking coffee results in a strong urge to urinate. This effect is due to the fact that coffee is a diuretic and promotes the excretion of fluids from your body. So, when you enjoy your daily ration of coffee, be sure to take in extra amounts of non-caffeinated beverages such as water or juice.

Moderation is also in vogue with coffee consumption since coffee can raise the level of chemicals associated with an increased risk of heart disease.

Last, if you regularly drink coffee hotter than 157 degrees, you could be at risk for a fourfold increase in the risk of cancer of the esophagus. Most restaurants, by the way, serve coffee between 170 to 190F.

Health Yourself

Unscrambling the Mystery of Eggs

Eating eggs two or three times a week has no negative effect on health and does not affect cholesterol levels for most people. In fact, researchers have found that eggs contain one-third less cholesterol than was previously thought. According to a report in the January 2001 issue of *RFN*, "The lowly but beloved egg may be emerging from the list of foods to avoid and could take its place along with good-for-you foods like tofu, beans, and lean meat." One good reason to endorse eggs is that the yolks contain lutein, a nutrient that may help prevent clogged arteries. Research findings reported in the medical journal *Circulation* indicated that higher blood levels of lutein were associated with less thickening of artery walls (*Allure Magazine* [*AM*], December 2001).

A single egg contains six grams of "very high quality" protein along with vitamins A, B-12, D, folate, thiamine, riboflavin, phosphorus, carotenoids, and zinc, all of which can have positive health benefits.

Researchers reporting in a 1999 volume of the *Journal of the American Medical Association* (*JAMA*) suggest that up to one egg a day is safe for the heart if you exercise, have normal blood pressure and cholesterol, and no family history of heart disease. You do the math. That's 365 eggs a year (over 12 dozen), and that's no yolk!

Yogurt – A Cultural Experience with a Touch of Sexy Blue

According to a review of several journal articles in *RFN* (October 2000), "Yogurt may be the ultimate health food by enhancing the immune response in those who eat it regularly."

Eating "live" or "activated" yogurt cultures regularly can improve your body's defenses against infection. Besides being an excellent source of calcium, yogurt has a positive effect on the immune system, which controls the body's responses against disease-causing bacteria. Adding low-fat yogurt to your breakfast choices can also supply you with some of the

Pantry Prevention

calcium you need to protect yourself against osteoporosis, the disease that thins your bones and results in painful and even deadly fractures.

Yogurt also contains bacteria that can help eliminate the other strains of bacteria known to trigger chronic migraine headaches, report Italian researchers in *MH* (September 2000).

Fresh Fruit

Adding fresh fruit such as blueberries or strawberries to your yogurt can increase your enjoyment as well as your health benefits. Research reported in the health section of the January 2000 edition of *AM* claims blueberries to be the most potent source of antioxidants in our food, and the report also notes other recent studies suggesting that blueberries may also help improve balance and coordination.

How are blueberries like sex? Tufts University researchers recently discovered that anthocyanins, the chemicals that give blueberries their color, increase the ability of brain cells to send and receive signals from other cells, resulting in improved mental function and enhanced memory. This report in *MH* (October 2001) noted that this same effect on brain function occurs with sexual activity. A more recent article says that blueberries can even have the same effect as the little blue prescription pill men take to improve their sexual functioning.

Bananas are also good for you. They contain high levels of vitamin B-6 that boost production of the brain chemical serotonin, resulting in a better mood, less stress, and more positive emotions.

Don't overlook oranges, either. Packed with vitamin C, one orange contains more than 100% of the daily requirement that, among other benefits, has been shown to reduce the risk of gallstones in women. Reducing gallstones could prevent several million operations a year and significantly lower health care costs.

Health Yourself

Experts recommend 250 to 500 milligrams of vitamin C a day to boost the body's immune system and fight off infections. According to the *UCBWL* (May 2000), "Many good studies show that vitamin C has potential benefits against cancer, heart disease, cataracts, and other disorders." Another group of medical researchers found vitamin C to be useful for younger patients with exercise-induced asthma, according to a 1998 report in the *UCBWL*.

Eight ounces of orange juice a day supplies the full daily requirement of vitamin C, but if you don't care for oranges or citrus fruit, you may soon be able to absorb vitamin C from your clothes! A Japanese company has developed a T-shirt made with fibers that turn into vitamin C when they make contact with your skin. According to a health columnist in the December 2001 issue of *Modern Maturity* (*MM*), the company is also developing vitamin rich underwear!

Besides vitamin C, oranges contain over 170 potent plant chemicals known as phytochemicals that have a wide array of positive effects. Doctors reported in *JAMA* (1999) that one extra serving per day of fruits or vegetables such as citrus fruits reduced the risk of stroke by 20%. Another study in Israel linked orange juice consumption to a decrease in LDL, the "bad" cholesterol, while Canadian researchers suggested that drinking three glasses of orange juice a day could raise your HDL, the "good" cholesterol.

Citrus fruits also contain limonene, a substance that stimulates the production of cancer-killing cells, and coumarins, natural blood thinners that help reduce blood clots and may also have effects that fight cancer.

Oranges are also sources of lutein and zeaxanthin, antioxidant chemicals important for maintaining the healthy function of your eyes and for reducing the risk of prostate cancer.

As I was growing up, whenever Uncle Russ visited we always had grapefruit on hand since that was all he ever ate for breakfast. He's still around and kicking in his seventies, thanks to the anti-oxidants and chemicals in grapefruit that reduce the risk of cancer and heart disease and boost the body's immune system. Back then, Uncle Russ didn't have to worry about the effects of grapefruit juice on his prescription medications, but today it's a different story. If you eat half a grapefruit or drink eight ounces of grapefruit juice, that's enough to

Pantry Prevention

have a serious effect on medications such as statins, the class of drugs prescribed to lower cholesterol. Grapefruit juice tends to increase the levels of statin drugs 5- to 15-fold, which could result in dangerous side effects.

Other medications that may interact with grapefruits and grapefruit juice include pain pills, allergy and asthma drugs, cancer drugs, heart medications, tranquilizers, and hormones. If you take any of these prescriptions and if you are a grapefruit fan like Uncle Russ, check with your doctor or pharmacist to see if there is any negative interaction between your medications and the grapefruit.

Water, Water Everywhere...

We often take this life-giving substance for granted, but water is not only necessary for our bodies' chemical reactions and processes, it also possesses some unexpected health benefits. Unfortunately, most of us don't drink enough water to keep our bodies supplied with the fluids we need to perform vital functions or to achieve the health benefits. Experts estimate that up to 75% of Americans are chronically dehydrated. Researchers have shown that drinking five eight-ounce glasses of water daily resulted in a decreased risk of deadly heart attacks in a group of patients who did not have a history of heart disease, stroke, or diabetes. Men who drank five or more glasses of water a day had a 51% decreased risk of fatal heart attacks compared to those men who drank fewer than two glasses a day. For women, there was a 35% reduction in risk for deadly heart attacks. Drinking five glasses of water daily also reduced the risk of having a killer stroke by 44%.

Men who drank more than two and a half liters of water a day had a nearly 50% lower incidence of bladder cancer compared to those who consumed only half as much water. Each additional cup of water daily reduced the risk by another seven percent, and the relationship between fluid intake and cancer prevention was as strong for smokers as for non-smokers. Smokers have a three- to five-fold higher rate of bladder cancers than non-smokers do, and thus they would benefit most from increasing their fluid intake or, better yet, from stopping smoking!

Health Yourself

Patients whose blood pressure drops too low, especially after a meal or with rapid position changes, may also benefit from drinking more water. However, researchers caution that drinking water can also raise blood pressure in those who already have elevated levels, so always be aware of your recent intake of water when checking your blood pressure.

Other possible benefits of five glasses a day include risk reduction for colon, bladder, and breast cancers. The same article in *Family Practice News* (*FPN*, October 1998) reported that five glasses of water a day can substantially lower the risk of a fatal stroke.

Drinking water 10 minutes before mealtime may also help you stay on your weight loss program. Thirst is often mistaken for hunger and may cause you to eat instead of replenishing your supply of liquids. When midnight hunger pangs strike, drinking a glass of water may make the craving disappear. If water isn't your cup of tea, you might want to try a glass of diet soda before a meal or when you feel the urge to snack. "Drinking soda can help quench your appetite as effectively as drinking milk or juice," notes a study from the University of Washington (*MH*, October 2002). Nutrition expert and author Dr. Jo Lichten assures us that the artificial sweeteners in diet sodas have proved to be safe and do not cause cancer or other serious health problems.

Almost half of Americans drink bottled water regularly. Bottled water may be no better than tap water, but it certainly is more expensive. In one study, researchers found that bacterial counts were higher in the commercially bottled water than in home tap water (*UCBWL*). Read the label carefully to determine the source of the bottled water, since many companies use regular tap water from the public water supply, and remember: "Evian" spelled backwards is "naïve."

Though you can substitute other beverages, consuming water is preferable to drinking liquids such as coffees, teas, and sodas. In fact, a study published in a medical journal revealed that bone fractures were linked to the consumption of carbonated beverages. Even physically active soda drinkers are at a higher risk for fractures. Experts believe that the high phosphorus content of sodas causes a chemical reaction that leads to bone loss.

Fiber

Many foods contain indigestible threads called fiber that provide special benefits such as protection from heart disease, stroke, diverticulitis, and diabetes. Fiber comes in two forms: soluble and insoluble. Soluble fibers dissolve in water and are easily absorbed from the intestine into the body. Oat bran products, beans, and psyllium contain the soluble type of fiber that helps lower cholesterol. Insoluble fibers are found in wheat and wheat bran products and remain inside the intestinal tract, where they undergo chemical changes that produce intestinal gas.

High fiber diets reduce many of the risk factors for heart disease, according to multiple research articles mentioned in *RFN* (2000). One of these was a Harvard University study that showed eating three or more servings of whole grain foods a day reduced heart attack risk 33% for women and 41% for men. Swedish researchers showed that patients whose diets had the highest cereal fiber content had the lowest rates of stomach cancer (*FPN* 2001).

Another Harvard study showed that those who had a daily intake of 24 grams of fiber were 57% less likely to develop high blood pressure than those who consumed only half that much fiber. (Check the nutrition label to see how much fiber is in each serving.) Another group of researchers found that for every five-gram increase in your daily intake of cereal fiber, there was a 37% decrease in the risk of heart disease (*RFN* 2000).

Scientists also found that eating at least five servings of fiber-rich fruits and vegetables daily produced a 31% decrease in stroke risk compared to those who ate few or no fruits and vegetables.

Feeling Your Oats

Once used only as animal food, oats have emerged as a beneficial dietary

Health Yourself

option for two-legged animals as well. Oats come from a whole-grain source rich in soluble fibers, one of which is beta glucan, a potent agent for reducing "bad" cholesterol, which can lead to heart disease.

Oat bran bread, which is high in fiber, resulted in better control of blood sugar for diabetics compared to white bread. In a study of women ages 40 to 65, results showed that those with the highest fiber intake had the lowest risk of developing diabetes.

Nearly 50% of all Americans over 60 years of age develop diverticulitis, an inflammatory condition of the large intestine that causes pain and abnormal bowel function. High fiber diets cut the risk of diverticulitis by 40%, while low fiber diets are a risk factor for developing this condition.

Weight loss experts recommend eating more high fiber foods, as they are low in fat and calories and tend to make you feel full and thus take the edge off hunger pangs. These foods also slow down the exit of food from the stomach, causing you to feel full earlier and longer, which may help decrease appetite and assist in weight loss. Dr. David L. Katz of Yale University Medical School reviewed the research on fiber and oats and found that an intake of five to 30 grams daily reduced food intake and hunger and produced weight loss that lasted up to a year. He also found that those who ate less than six grams of fiber daily weighed eight pounds more than those who consumed more than 11 grams of dietary fiber daily. In another three studies involving 182 overweight patients placed on different diets, those who incorporated oat-bran biscuits into their daily diet were more successful at losing weight.

Oats are rich in phytochemicals that lower the risk of heart disease and they can also help diabetics control blood sugar levels by improving the body's sensitivity to natural insulin.

Researchers in Minnesota monitored the eating habits of nearly 300 teenagers and found that those who ate the most whole grains were the leanest and had the least insulin resistance, a strong predictor of future heart disease, strokes, and diabetes (*Prevention Magazine* [*PM*], May 2002). Nutrition experts recommend using non-sugared fiber cereals such as

Pantry Prevention

Cheerios, Wheaties, and Shredded Wheat for snacks, and kids, teens, and adults can also increase their fiber intake with enjoyable options such as air-popped or low fat microwave popcorn, whole wheat pasta, or whole wheat English muffins.

See the chart below for detailed nutritional information on cereals that are good sources of oats and fiber.

PRODUCT	CALORIES	FAT (g)	% CALORIES FROM FAT	FIBER (g)
GOOD SOURCES OF OATS				
Kellogg's Cracklin' Oat Bran Cereal, 3/4 cup (2 oz)	190	7	33	6
Quaker Toasted Oatmeal Cereal, 1 cup (2 oz)	190	2.5	12	3
MultiGrain Cheerios, 1 cup (1 oz)	110	1	8	3
Health Valley Oat Bran O's Cereal, 3/4 cup (1 oz)	100	0	0	3
Healthy Choice Low-Fat Granola, 2/3 cup (2 oz)	220	3	12	3
Matthew's Oat Bran Bread, 1 slice	60	1	15	2
QUESTIONABLE SOURCES				
Nabisco Oatmeal Cookies, 1	80	3	34	0
Pennysticks Oat Bran Pretzel Nuggets, 1 oz	120	2	15	1
Kellogg's NutriGrain Cereal Bar, 1 bar (1.3 oz)	140	3	19	1
Nabisco Harvest Crisps, 5-Grain (with rolled oats), 1 oz	130	3.5	24	1

The American Heart Association recommends a daily intake of 25 to 35 grams of fiber. Most Americans eat less than half that amount, so there's room for improvement. Take the advice of the American Heart Association and prescribe yourself more fiber! See the chart on the following page for help in figuring out how much fiber is in certain foods.

Health Yourself

COMPARISON OF FOODS AND THEIR FIBER AMOUNTS

Food labels will list the amount of total dietary fiber but will not always list the soluble fiber amount. Here's the soluble fiber content of some common foods:

FOOD	AMOUNT	DIETARY FIBER (grams)	SOLUBLE FIBER (grams)
BREAD	**1 SLICE**		
White		0.6	0.3
Whole wheat		2.0	0.3
Oatmeal		1.1	0.6
Rye		1.5	0.8
CEREAL	**1 CUP**		
Crispy rice		0.3	0.1
Corn flakes		0.8	0.1
Hot creamy wheat		0.9	0.4
Toasted oatmeal squares		3.0	0.9
Oatmeal, instant	1 pouch	3.0	1.0
Oatmeal, old-fashioned and quick		4.0	2.0
FRUIT			
Apple juice	1/2 cup	0.2	0.0
Banana, fresh	1 medium	2.8	0.8
Strawberries	1 cup	3.3	0.9
Apple, with skin	1 medium	3.8	1.0
Orange	1 medium	3.1	1.8
Blackberries	1 cup	7.6	1.4
DRIED BEANS	**1/2 CUP**		
Pinto, cooked from dried		7.4	1.9
Navy, cooked from dried		5.8	2.2
Kidney, cooked from dried		5.7	2.8
VEGETABLES	**1 CUP**		
Tomato, raw, cooked from frozen		2.0	0.2
Carrots, raw		3.3	1.7
Broccoli, cooked from frozen		5.5	2.8

Source: Spiller, G.A.: *CRC Handbook of Dietary Fiber in Human Nutrition*, 3rd Edition. CRC Press, Boca Raton, Florida, 2001.

Rice Is Nice

Fiber-rich rice bran can lower cholesterol, according to recent research reported in *UCBWL* (August 2000). After brown rice is milled to become white rice, the leftovers are the rice bran. You can enjoy it by sprinkling it on cereal, salads, and yogurt or by adding it to muffins, breads, and cakes. Rice bran also contains unsaturated oils that provide additional cholesterol-lowering effects.

Pantry Prevention

The chart below, published in a prestigious medical journal, can help you find enjoyable ways to increase your daily fiber intake and experience the positive health benefits mentioned earlier.

SAMPLE MENUS FOR INCREASING DIETARY FIBER AND SOLUBLE FIBER

With small changes, the dietary fiber content of the following diet doubled and the soluble fiber content tripled. The • marks the food changes that increased the fiber.

STANDARD DIET	HIGH-FIBER DIET
24 grams dietary fiber, 8 grams soluble fiber	50 grams dietary fiber, 25 grams soluble fiber
BREAKFAST	
Orange juice	• Orange sections
White grits	• Oatmeal
Egg substitute	Scrambled egg
Olive oil	Olive oil
Decaffeinated coffee	Decaffeinated coffee
LUNCH	
Ham	Ham
Mayonnaise	Mayonnaise
Iceberg lettuce	Iceberg lettuce
Fresh tomato	Fresh tomato
Low-sodium bread	• Whole-wheat bread
Corn (canned)	Corn (canned)
Cider (vinegar)	• Green peas (canned)
Dehydrated onion	Dehydrated onion
Olive oil	Olive oil
Fresh green pepper	Fresh green pepper
Fresh celery	Fresh celery
Instant tea	Instant tea
Oatmeal raisin cookie	
DINNER	
Chicken breast (skinned)	Chicken breast (skinned)
Bran flakes	Bran flakes
Low-sodium bread	• Oat bran
Parmesan cheese	Parmesan cheese
Whole egg	Egg substitute
Tomato (canned)	Tomato (canned)
Low-fat cheese	Low-fat cheese
Spaghetti	Spaghetti
Green beans	• Zucchini
Olive oil	Olive oil
Whole-wheat bread	Whole-wheat bread
Graham crackers	• Fresh peaches
Instant tea	Instant tea
BEDTIME SNACK	
Mozzarella cheese	• Fruit cocktail (canned)
Low-sodium bread	• Cherries (canned)
Pineapple juice	• Granola

Source: Beneficial effects of high dietary fiber intake in patients with type 2 diabetes melitus. NEJM 342 (19:1392-1398), 2000

Health Yourself

Life after Breakfast

After breakfast we traditionally have at least two meals to get us through the rest of the day, but some researchers recommend eating more frequent smaller meals rather than three larger ones. I call this pattern of eating "grazing," and it can yield positive health benefits. Specifically, eating small frequent meals is better for cholesterol levels than eating the traditional "three square meals a day," according to an article in the *British Medical Journal* (*AFP*, May 2002). Grazing can also result in more consistent blood sugar levels during the day and can decrease uncomfortable hunger pangs. Skipping meals may seem like a smart strategy for losing weight, but it often has the opposite effect, says Jo Ann Hattner, R.D., of the American Dietetic Association. She recommends eating "at least every four hours" to avoid becoming excessively hungry and giving way to cravings and urges. (*Self* magazine, October 2002).

While I was visiting the Provence region of southern France to educate a group of doctors about PRO-vention not too long ago, I noticed very few overweight people in the cities and villages. During my weeklong stay I ate the bulk of my meals at local restaurants that offered mostly regional dishes characteristic of the "Mediterranean Diet." I also noticed that regular restaurants, bistros, and brasseries vastly outnumbered the fast food outlets we see in America. As Uncle Doo-Dad said, "I don't consider snails fast food."

When I returned home, I researched the components of the Mediterranean diet and found it to have many beneficial effects besides promoting a healthy weight. In other parts of the world this diet is called the Okinawan diet.

According to the *Johns Hopkins Medical Letter* (*JHML*, November 2001), residents of Okinawa, an island located in the Pacific Ocean between Japan and Taiwan, boast several incredible health claims. Researchers have found Okinawa to have the highest concentration of people over 100 years old and the longest disability-free life span in the world. Okinawans have such a low incidence of breast and prostate cancer that screening tests for the diseases are unnecessary. Scientists agree that dietary habits of the

Pantry Prevention

Okinawans account for most of these health benefits. Like the Mediterranean diet, the Okinawan menu is extremely low in fats, which account for less than 25% of the total calories for a day, and most of these fat calories are of the healthier unsaturated variety. Fat calories, mostly of the more dangerous saturated variety of fats, make up 35% of the average American diet! Let's see what we can learn from our neighbors in the Okinawan and Mediterranean regions.

In Okinawa, an average day's food intake consists of seven servings of fruits and vegetables, another seven helpings of whole grains such as brown rice and noodles, and at least two servings of soy in the form of miso, tofu, or soybeans. Small amounts of meat, fish, and dairy products round out the typical Okinawan diet. American patients who followed a Mediterranean diet experienced similar health benefits. After having a heart attack, they reduced their risk of dying by 40% over the next six years. Let's look at the food that makes up the "Mediterranean Diet."

Olive Oil

A staple of the Mediterranean diet, olive oil is often used in cooking and salads and can add more than just flavor to your life. This tasty liquid not only protects you against heart disease, it may also lower your chances of developing rheumatoid arthritis, a painful and crippling condition caused by inflammation of the joints. Some patients with mild to moderate high blood pressure whose main source of dietary fat was olive oil were able to reduce their daily dose of blood pressure medications by 48% while nearly one-fourth of the patients were able to discontinue their blood pressure medications completely, according to research reported in a 2000 issue of *Hippocrates* magazine.

Adding olive oil to your meals makes good sense, but remember it has 100 calories per teaspoon, and only one-third of your total calories should come from fat. *UCBWL* editors reviewed the results of 14 important studies about olive oil and cholesterol and reported their findings in the February 1999 issue. They came to the conclusion that "If your chief concern is lowering blood cholesterol, you have nothing to gain by choosing olive oil over…oils such as corn or soybean." Researchers caution that olive oil is not a magic bullet and that while it has positive health benefits, it "won't compensate for an unhealthy diet."

Fruits and Veggies

Fruits and vegetables are abundant in the Mediterranean diet. Apples, citrus fruits, apricots, berries, prunes, cabbages, sweet potatoes, and Brussels sprouts all contain high levels of pectin, a special kind of fiber that lowers both overall cholesterol and LDL, "bad" cholesterol, an effect that can reduce heart disease and stroke.

Broccoli, grown in Italy since ancient Roman times (and disparaged by former President G. H. Bush), contains more vitamin C in a one-cup serving than there is in a whole orange! This cruciferous (crunchy) vegetable is packed with other beneficial nutrients such as potassium, vitamin K, and folic acid and is an excellent source of fiber. When broccoli passes through the digestive tract, it also produces high levels of a cancer-fighting chemical. Maybe that's why a high intake of cruciferous vegetables like broccoli and cabbage significantly reduces the risk of bladder cancer in people who never smoked. Non-smoking men who ate more than five servings a week had more than a 50% reduction of risk for bladder cancer compared to those who ate only one serving a week.

Broccoli also contains chemicals that affect the body's production of the female hormone estrogen, stimulating the manufacture of the benign forms of estrogen that are not associated with breast cancer.

One cup of broccoli has fewer than 50 calories and *no* fats or cholesterol if you use lemon juice instead of butter to add a little zing. (See the section on margarine and butter below.)

Black beans, kidney beans, and lima beans are also excellent sources of soluble fiber, a potent agent for reducing cholesterol levels in the bloodstream. Eating four ounces of these types of beans a day can lower overall

Pantry Prevention

cholesterol as well as LDL or "bad" cholesterol. One recent study found that eating beans and peanuts, a food group known as "legumes," four times a week resulted in nearly 20% less coronary artery disease (the cause of heart attacks) and a nearly 10% decrease in overall cardiovascular risk compared to those who ate these foods only once a week.

Beans are also high in zinc, a mineral that is important to your immune system and helps shorten the duration of colds.

Tomatoes are plentiful in the Mediterranean diet, and adding this tasty fruit to your daily menu can give you some great health benefits due to nutrients such as vitamin C, a potent antioxidant that soaks up free radicals – the dangerous chemicals that can cause DNA mutations and lead to cancer.

Eating tomatoes seven times a week cuts the risk of prostate, lung, and stomach cancer in half compared to those who eat them only once a week, according to Harvard Medical School researcher Dr. Edward Giovannuci. Chemicals called lycopenes are responsible for this cancer-fighting activity and have been shown to have a lesser protective effect against cancers of the pancreas, colon, esophagus, mouth, breast, and cervix. In 1999 experts at the National Cancer Institute reviewed 72 different research projects and found that tomato intake reduced cancer in 57 studies, 35 of which were statistically insignificant, with another 15 studies inconclusive. Tomatoes are also rich in p-coumaric acid and chlorogenic acid, chemicals that act as scavengers and help remove dangerous substances from the body. Green peppers, strawberries, and carrots also contain these scavenger-like chemicals.

If you like concentrated or processed forms of tomatoes such as ketchup, salsa, and tomato sauce you're in luck! These forms of tomatoes contain more active and more effective forms of lycopenes than the tomatoes picked fresh from the vine.

You can also get the beneficial effects of lycopenes from eating watermelon, apricots, pink grapefruit, red peppers, and carrots, so why not add a colorful array of vegetables and fruits to your diet?

Health Yourself

Any discussion of the Mediterranean region diet must mention grapes. A little later on we will see how grapes are used to make heart-healthy wines, but for now, let's focus on some of the other positive health aspects of these tasty morsels. Grapes are loaded with ellagic acid, a chemical that blocks the body's production of enzymes that cancer cells require to function and grow. Inside the grape we also find phenols, which prevent blood clots from forming, and reservatrol, a natural fungus killer that slows the accumulation of bad cholesterol. If you want to enjoy the benefits of grapes without indulging in alcohol, drinking grape juice can be an excellent source.

Some Like It Hot!

Capsaicin, the chemical found in several varieties of peppers, helps neutralize cancer-causing chemicals called nitrosamines. The hotter the peppers, the higher the level of capsaicin they contain. Jalapeno peppers and Thai peppers are the hottest varieties and offer the most protection. Capsaicin is also used as a cream to rub on the skin to relieve arthritis pains, but be sure to wash the cream off your hands so you won't burn your eyes or other sensitive areas. Eating jalapeno nachos with your fingers can prevent cancer and treat arthritis all at the same time!

The Main Courses

Fish dishes are often the main course in the Mediterranean and Okinawan diets. Fatty fish such as salmon are rich in omega-3 fats that have positive effects on the heart and comprise a substantial portion of our brain cells. Researchers have found that people who consume large amounts of fatty fish have much lower rates of depression than those who eat less seafood. Duke University scientists found that young women with cholesterol levels less than 160 were more likely to experience depression than their counterparts who had normal or elevated cholesterol levels. Researchers attribute the depression to the low levels of omega-3 fatty acids that help the cholesterol circulate throughout the body.

Pantry Prevention

One serving of fatty fish per week can also reduce the risk of heart attack by 50 to 70%, according to *JAMA* (December, 2002). Experts at the U.S. Department of Veteran Affairs determined that the higher levels of fat and protein found in fatty fish helped protect against the memory loss associated with stroke.

Omega-3 fish oils can also help relieve menstrual cramps as effectively as over- the-counter medications such as ibuprofen (*Self* magazine, August 2001). This study from Denmark showed that women who ate the most fish had a lower occurrence of menstrual cramps. Another study showed that teenage girls experienced relief of premenstrual syndrome (PMS) from either taking 1.8 grams of omega-3 fish oil tablets daily for three months or eating three ounces of salmon a day.

Enjoying salmon, mackerel, tuna, and bluefish results in high levels of omega-3 fatty acids that lower cholesterol and thus offer protection against heart disease. For this reason, the American Heart Association recommends eating salmon or tuna at least twice a week to protect against heart disease, our number-one killer.

Numerous studies also show that patients with rheumatoid arthritis have less fatigue and joint stiffness when they consume the omega-3 fish oil, especially early in the disease process. Likewise, more than half of patients with irritable bowel syndrome and Crohn's disease (inflammation of the bowel) experienced relief of symptoms while taking omega-3 with their prescribed medication.

These studies also show that women who ate fish were 22% less likely to have a stroke than women who ate fish only once a month. According to this *JAMA* study reported in *Family Practice News* (September 2002), eating fish five times a week cut the risk of stroke in half.

Omega-3 fatty acids also occur in wild game, avocados, canola oil, and nuts such as almonds and walnuts.

Health Yourself

Selenium: Mineral Rights

Those finned critters that swim are also excellent sources of selenium, a trace mineral known to be a mood elevator. A USDA study found that men who took extra selenium in their meals reported feeling happier at the end of the day than those who did not receive the extra helping of the supplement. You can also get high levels of selenium when you enjoy a lean sirloin steak; the trace mineral is also found in nuts and oatmeal.

Another recent study showed that taking in 200 micrograms of selenium daily lowered the risk of prostate, lung, and colorectal cancer by 45 to 63%. Selenium may also offer protection against lung and liver cancers, but experts also caution that the trace mineral is toxic in high doses. Dr. Gerald Combs Jr. of Cornell University made a strong statement about the powers of selenium: "There is perhaps no more extensive body of evidence for the cancer-preventive potential of a normal dietary component than there is for selenium."

"The Meat of the Matter"

If you prefer red meats such as beef, pork, and lamb, go for it! While eating these red meats has been linked to colon and prostate cancers, experts are unsure how much of the effect is due to the fat content or the cancer-causing chemicals that form when protein is cooked at a high temperature. These meats are excellent sources of protein, vitamins, and zinc as well as other important nutrients. Here are some tips to help you enjoy your favorite red meats safely:

- Choose low-fat cuts of meat.
- Use small portions.
- Drain off fat.
- Bake and broil rather than char or fry.
- Marinating before cooking reduces the amount of cancer-causing chemicals (heterocyclic amines) by 92 to 99%.

Pantry Prevention

- Use vinegar, olive oil, and lemon juice to marinate your favorite meat.

- When preparing chicken, you can reduce the fat content by 75% and cut the total calories in half by removing the skin before cooking. Dark-meat chicken has two to three times as much fat as a skinless chicken breast and 25% more calories. Some lean cuts of beef and pork have the same fat per ounce as skinless dark-meat chicken.

  (Note: Even though not all of these foods are included in the Mediterranean diet, they can still be healthy and enjoyable additions to your meals.)

The Shell Game

Choosing clams and oysters from the menu can help your body fight off dangerous germs and bacteria by supplying high levels of zinc to your white blood cells, your body's main line of defense. A three-ounce serving of oysters contains five times the recommended daily intake of zinc. Toss some of these shellfish into soup or pasta sauce or create a "defensive dip" by mixing them with plain yogurt or low-fat sour cream.

Vegging Out

Butternut squash is so rich in beta carotene, a chemical compound that your body converts into vitamin A, that just one cup of this winter favorite supplies your daily need for vitamin A which, in turn, fortifies your body's protective tissues. Nutrition expert Dr. Liz Applegate, the nutritional columnist of *RW*, makes a butternut squash casserole at least once a week in the winter and says she "usually remains cold-free."

Garlic and onions may ward off more than evil spirits and friends, according to clinical nutritionists such as Dr. Applegate. Onions, leeks, and garlic are members of the allium family of vegetables and are chock-full of the antioxidant querectin that protects against bacterial infections and even helps fight cancer. Only the chopped and freeze-dried forms of garlic offer heart protection; taking garlic supplements does not provide the same level of protection. A good rule to remember is, "If it doesn't give you garlic breath, it probably won't protect you."

Health Yourself

By the way, European researchers gave people artichoke extract twice a day before meals and found that LDL cholesterol levels dropped along with total cholesterol levels. Eating the real thing ought to produce the same results.

The Skin Game

People who have the lowest amount of fats in their diets have healthier skin than those who indulge more heavily in fatty foods. Indeed, low-fat diets result in less risk of skin cancer and fewer wrinkles. High intake of vegetables, olive oil, fish, and legumes results in smoother, younger looking skin compared to diets dominated by meat and dairy products, resulting in the most wrinkling (*Journal of the American College of Nutrition*, 2001).

In the mid-1990s researchers at Baylor College of Medicine showed that skin cancer patients who were put on a low-fat diet (less than 20% of total calories from fat) developed only one-third as many tumors and lesions as those whose diet had 38% of its calories from fat. A low-fat diet that includes at least five servings of fruits and vegetables daily protects against pre-cancerous skin problems (actinic keratoses) as well as against actual skin cancers.

Migraine patients who limited their fat intake to 20 grams per day likewise reduced their frequency of headaches by 70%, reduced the intensity of their pain by 68%, and *shortened* the length of their headaches by 74%.

Bone Up with Protein

Elderly people who increase their protein intake may benefit from a decreased risk of osteoporosis. In a recent study published in the *Journal of Bone and Mineral Research,* those elderly people who consumed the least amount of protein had more bone loss than those who consumed a higher level of protein. Protein intake showed a benefit regardless of the person's age, weight, smoking habits, calcium intake, or estrogen. Excellent sources of protein include fish, poultry, lean cuts of red meat, and lentils.

Pantry Prevention

Summer Treat (and a Treatment for Sinus Trouble)

Researchers in the Netherlands found that sinus sufferers are deficient in glutathione, an antioxidant chemical found in watermelons, grapefruit, oranges, broccoli, asparagus, peaches, and potatoes.

Your respiratory tract is lined with cells that need glutathione to balance out the free radicals that cause inflammation and lead to disease. Chicken soup, the traditional home remedy, may actually provide relief by supplying cysteine (found in chicken meat), which the body uses to manufacture glutathione.

The Eyes Have It

Researchers at Florida International University in Miami found that eating fruits and vegetables rich in lutein and zeaxanthin may reduce the risk of age-related macular degeneration, the main cause of vision loss in people over 50. You get these important chemicals from eating broccoli, corn, squash, and dark green leafy vegetables like spinach. If you like Mexican food, look for spinach enchiladas and corn tortillas on the menu. If you are a burger or sandwich fan, top your creation with spinach instead of lettuce.

Two additional large studies suggest a lower risk of cataracts for people who eat corn, spinach, pumpkin, zucchini, yellow squash, red grapes, and green peas.

Breadbasket Beats the Blues

Whole grain foods such as cereals, breads, and pastas not only supply the high levels of energy your body needs for fuel, they also start a series of chemical reactions that lead to a higher level of serotonin in your brain, resulting in an improved mood. Nutritional experts recommend 8 to 12 servings of whole grain products per day.

Health Yourself

Butter Yourself Up and Your Cholesterol Down

If you butter up your bread or broccoli using canola oil margarines such as Benecol or Take Control, you can lower your cholesterol like the 600 heart attack patients in a research study who decreased their risk of a second heart attack by 70%. Researchers suspect, but have yet to prove, that using this special margarine could also reduce the risk of a first heart attack by virtue of its ability to lower levels of LDL ("bad" cholesterol) by 7 to 10%, even in patients with normal cholesterol levels (*FPN*, June 1999). Look for these products in the dairy case at your local supermarket.

The recommended intake of three servings of an ounce and a half per day will cost about five dollars a week. If the expense doesn't give you a heart attack, these products may be a positive addition to your heart-healthy diet. Even at their high price, they are cheaper than the traditional cholesterol-lowering drugs and have fewer serious side effects (*UCBWL*, August 1999).

Soup to Nuts

Whenever my brothers or I had to stay home from school with a cold, flu, or sore throat, my mother always fed us the same array of foods that we all still associate with being sick. I'm sure your mothers and grandmothers did the same thing. Mother always gave us Jell-O, grape juice, Seven-up, ginger ale, and chicken noodle soup. Recent research confirms that chicken soup is not only a good name for a book, it also has strong antibacterial properties that have earned it the nickname "Maternal Penicillin." The ingredients in chicken soup boost the effectiveness of the white blood cells as they fight off infection-causing bacteria such as upper respiratory infections (*Chest* medical journal, 2000).

Nuts to You!

Then there are nuts. Researchers have found that women who eat more than five ounces (one-half cup) of nuts per week have a 35% lower risk of

Pantry Prevention

heart disease than those women who eat few or no nuts (*AFP*, April 1999). The obvious conclusion is, "Nuts to you, Ladies!" Another study of 31,000 people in California determined that eating peanuts or other nuts five times a week cut their heart disease risk by half. Eating nuts instead of meats and cheese replaces saturated fats (dangerous fats) with monosaturated or polyunsaturated fats (good fats) that act to lower cholesterol. Nuts also contain other chemicals that block your body's ability to absorb cholesterol through your intestine. Two to four ounces of nuts daily resulted in a four percent reduction in cholesterol, which in turn yields an eight percent reduction in the risk of heart disease (*BMJ*, 1998; *AFP*, April 1999; *UCBWL*, April 1999).

So enjoy that peanut butter: it's rich in folate and Vitamin E, which are both important to heart health.

Caution: nuts contain up to 200 calories per ounce and are high in fat, containing 14 to 19 grams per ounce, so enjoy them in moderation. Watch out for the high salt (sodium) content if you are concerned about high blood pressure or congestive heart failure.

Just for fun, test your degree of nuttiness by taking the following "Nutty Quiz" from *UCBWL*'s April 1999 issue:

Nutty Quiz

See if you can match each nut to its special trait.

1. Highest in fat
2. Only low-fat nut; rich in fiber
3. Rich in vitamin B-6 and heart-healthy oil
4. Rich in vitamin E and folic acid
5. Rich in selenium
6. Not true nuts, but legumes
7. Rich in copper, iron, and folic acid
8. Rich in calcium, vitamin E, and fiber

(a) almonds
(b) brazil nuts
(c) cashews
(d) chestnuts
(e) hazelnuts
(f) macadamia
(g) peanuts
(h) walnuts

Answers: 1(f), 2 (d), 3 (h), 4 (e), 5 (b), 6 (g), 7 (c), 8 (a)

Health Yourself

DASH Your Way to Health

Medical experts tested various diets for their ability to lower blood pressure and prevent heart attacks and strokes. This project was known as the Dietary Approach to Stop Hypertension, or DASH, study. In this trial, researchers compared the effects of three diets: the average American diet, a diet high in fruits and vegetables, and the DASH diet, which was even higher in fruits, vegetables, and low-fat dairy products and low in saturated fats and cholesterol.

Patients on this diet lowered their blood pressure significantly and experienced other health-related benefits as well. For example, gynecology specialists found that women who went on a high fiber vegetarian diet had significant reductions in their menstrual pain and PMS symptoms (*FPN*, July 2000).

The following chart shows the basics of the DASH diet.

DOING THE DASH
The DASH eating plan below is based on a 2,000 calorie-a-day diet.

Food group	Daily servings	Foods and serving sizes	Other foods	Nutrients for blood pressure
Grains & grain products	7-8 a day	1/2 cup oatmeal, 1 oz whole grain ready-to-eat cereal, 1 slice whole wheat bread	whole-wheat pita bread, whole wheat English muffin, popcorn, bagel	fiber, magnesium
Vegetables	4-5 a day	6 oz vegetable juice, 1/2 cup cooked vegetables, 1 cup raw leafy green vegetables	broccoli, carrots, collard greens, green peas, potatoes, squash, tomatoes, sweet potatoes	fiber, magnesium, potassium
Fruits	4-5 a day	6 oz fruit juice, 1 medium fruit, 1/2 cup dried fruit, 1/2 cup fresh, frozen, or canned fruit	apricots, bananas, dates, grapes, oranges, grapefruit, mangoes, melons, peaches, pineapples, prunes, strawberries	fiber, magnesium, potassium
Low-fat or fat free dairy foods	2-3 a day	8 oz skim or low-fat milk, 1 cup low-fat yogurt, 1 1/2 oz low-fat cheese	low-fat buttermilk, fat-free regular or frozen yogurt, fat-free cheese	calcium, protein
Meats, poultry, and fish	No more than 2 a day	3 oz cooked meat, poultry or fish	lean meat trimmed of fat, skinless poultry	magnesium
Nuts, seeds and dry beans	4-5 a week	1/3 cup or 1 1/2 oz nuts, 2 Tbsp or 1/2 oz seeds, 1/2 cup cooked dry beans	almonds, filberts, mixed nuts, peanuts, walnuts, sunflower seeds, kidney beans, lentils, peas	fiber, magnesium, potassium
Fat and oils	2-3 a day	1 tsp soft margarine, 1 Tbsp low-fat mayonnaise, 2 Tbsp light salad dressing, 1 tsp vegetable oil	olive, corn, canola, or safflower oil	DASH diet is low in fat

Pantry Prevention

An Apple a Day

Scientists at Cornell University reported in *Nature* that apples contain chemicals that stop the growth of colon and liver cancer cells in laboratory test tubes. These researchers claim that "Eating fruits and vegetables is better than taking a vitamin pill."

If Pain's the Pits, Try Cherries

Cherry growers in Michigan have long known that a handful of the tart fruit can ease the pain of arthritis and gout. Researchers from Michigan State University checked out the claim and found that cherries contain chemicals called anthocyanins that give them their red color and also act as antioxidants that protect against cancer and heart disease. This interesting chemical also reduced inflammation even better than aspirin. Blueberries, strawberries, and raspberries contain the same chemicals and may also be useful as pain relievers.

Soy – The Beans Have It; the Supplements Don't

25 grams of soy protein daily may reduce the risk of heart attack by improving cholesterol profiles, according to evidence presented to the Food and Drug Administration. Researchers from Tufts University found that soybean oil and margarine lowered levels of LDL ("bad" cholesterol) that are associated with increased risk of heart attacks (*NEJM*, 1999).

Soy foods also contain chemicals resembling the female hormone estrogen. These chemicals have been associated with reducing cancers of the colon, breast, uterus, and prostate and also reduce osteoporosis and menopausal symptoms such as hot flashes (*Patient Care*, December 2000). One researcher notes that Japanese women have a very high intake of soy and don't even have a word in their language for hot flashes. Two cups of soymilk, or four ounces of tofu daily, provide the health benefits (*RFN*, April 2000).

Health Yourself

Here's a list of some of the ways you can enjoy the soy!

- Use unflavored soymilk in cream-based soups.
- Use vanilla-flavored soymilk in milkshakes, morning coffee, or on your cereal.
- Use half soy protein and half meat when making tacos or casseroles.
- Use soy protein in spaghetti sauce, meat loaf, and sloppy joes.

(*RW*, April 2001)

In addition, soy cheese can be substituted for any form of spreadable cheese and can be used as a pizza topping, while soy flour can be used in place of regular flour in baking.

Soy nuts, one of my favorite snacks, come in a variety of spices and flavors. Send an e-mail request to my website at **www.healthyourselves.com** and I'll tell you my secret source of these great snacks.

Soy milk is lactose free and available in several flavors, but since I haven't found one I like yet, I'm sticking to nuts.

Last, tofu serves as a soybean curd dish that can be a cheese substitute in dips.

Caution: Soy supplements in the form of capsules and pills don't confer the same benefits as eating the food sources and are potentially dangerous at levels over 100 milligrams per day.

The Buzz on Honey

When you substitute honey for sugar, you are taking advantage of the powerful antioxidant properties that may help protect you from heart disease. University of Illinois researcher Dr. Nicki Engseth says, "Honey is right in line with strawberries and apples in overall antioxidant effect."

Experts at the University of Memphis recommend three tablespoons of honey, plain or in tea, an hour before starting your exercise. Dr. Conrad Earnest says, "Honey affects blood sugar levels more mildly than other

Pantry Prevention

sweets such as soda and jelly beans, providing a steady flow of energy during a long workout."

Got Milk?

Drinking milk may decrease your risk of colon cancer, according to Harvard University researchers. They found that men whose diets included 700 to 900 milligrams of calcium daily were up to 50% less likely to develop some forms of colon cancer than men whose diets had only 500 milligrams of calcium daily.

You can also help preserve your teeth by strengthening your gums with calcium. Men who consumed more than 800 milligrams of calcium daily had half the risk of gum disease as those men who consumed 500 milligrams or less of calcium per day (*MH*, October 2002).

Graze Away

A study published in the *British Medical Journal* (*BMJ*) showed that eating small frequent meals results in better cholesterol levels than eating the traditional three square meals a day. According to these researchers, the more often you eat, the lower your cholesterol level (*AFP*, May 2002).

Nutritional expert Jo Ann Hattner also recommends grazing as part of a successful weight loss regimen. She says that eating at least every four hours keeps you from becoming "frantically hungry" and reduces hunger cravings (*Self* magazine, October 2002).

Rewind the Aging Process

Adding the following five foods to your diet can reverse the effects of aging, according to *MH* (October 2002):

1. Sunflower seeds have the highest natural vitamin E content of any food around. According to Dr. Barry Swanson, professor of food science at

Health Yourself

Washington State University, "Vitamin E is one of the most important nutrients around for looking younger." Dr. Branson says, "No antioxidant is more effective at fighting the aging effects of free radicals." I guess that's why baseball players look so young.

2. Those men who ate the most leafy green vegetables and beans had the fewest wrinkles on their skin, thanks to the chemicals that help prevent and repair wear and tear on your skin cells as they age.

3. Grape juice contains chemicals that keep your skin flexible and elastic.

4. Sweet potatoes may help fight sun damage to your skin. European researchers found that pigments from foods rich in beta carotene, like sweet potatoes and carrots, can build up a protective layer in your skin, helping to prevent damage from ultraviolet rays.

5. Cheese can protect your teeth, according to Dr. Matthew Messina, spokesman for the American Dental Association. Dr. Messina says cheese provides calcium that keeps your teeth strong. He also says, "Eating cheese can lower the levels of bacteria in your mouth and keep your teeth clean and cavity free." Two servings of block cheese every week gives you the benefits.

Stop Browsing the Fridge and Start Browsing the Net

Web resources for dietary information include the following:

DASH Diet at http:// www.nhlbi.nih.gov/health/public/heart/hbp/dash, Mediterranean Diet at http://nutrition.about.com/health/nutrition/cs/mediterraneandiet, and American Dietetic Association at http://www.eatright.org/healthy/.

Candy Is Dandy...

About now you are probably wondering when we get to the good parts about prescribing candy, booze, and sex. Here's the first part of the best prescription you ever had: candy and chocolate! Depending on your overall medical condition and health status, you might want to include a moderate amount of sweets and candy in your personal PRO-vention plan. Recently, researchers studied almost 8,000 male graduates of Harvard University and found that chocolate and candy eaters live almost a year longer than those who abstain. Those who averaged one to three candy bars a month had a 36% lower risk of death compared to non-candy eaters.

Pantry Prevention

Even those who had a "heavy" intake of three or more sweets per week still enjoyed a 16% lower risk of death than those who almost never ate candy.

Chocolate contains chemicals that protect against heart disease and cancer, and cocoa contains substances that prevent dental plaque and gum disease by killing germs in the mouth. Chocolate appears to be less damaging to the teeth than other foods containing the same amount of sugar. One day, your dentist may even recommend brushing your teeth with chocolate toothpaste! A research study from Osaka University in Japan showed that an extract from the cocoa bean husk used to make chocolate had an antibacterial effect on the mouth and was effective in fighting plaque and other damaging substances (*AFP*).

One and a half ounces of chocolate also contains the same amount of phenols as a glass of red wine. Phenols have the same properties as antioxidants, preventing toxic substances from building up in the bloodstream and blocking circulation to vital organs such as the heart and brain. The author who reviewed the research article in *MBHN* says, "Perhaps it's not the phenols at all. Maybe it's the celebration of a special treat that boosts mood and results in a longer life" (*BMJ*, 1998; reported in *MBHN*, Vol. VIII, No. 1, 1999).

Chocolate and sweets may also have a use in relieving temporary pain. Canadian researchers observed that giving infants something sweet to suck on helped reduce the pain of medical procedures such as drawing blood and circumcision. The researchers tried the same approach on adults and found they, too, had a higher threshold for pain when they were tasting something sweet at the same time.

Chocolate is a very dense source of calories and saturated fat but in moderation can be a luscious addition to a healthy diet. Most of the problems with chocolate are due to what we mix with it. Nuts, cream, and coconut increase the caloric and fat content; chocolate by itself is a plant product derived from cocoa beans and is naturally free of cholesterol. Remember: if it doesn't have parents, it can't have cholesterol.

By the way, dermatologists now tell us there is no link between chocolate and acne. Thanks a lot. I gave up chocolate for two years as a teenager thinking it would improve my complexion!

Health Yourself

Caution: chocolate may aggravate headaches and heartburn in certain sensitive individuals. And when it comes to partaking of chocolate and sweets, remember: "More is not necessarily better."

...But Liquor Is Quicker

Here's the second installment of the candy, booze, and sex prescription. On my European sojourns, I noticed wine and alcohol to be an integral part of the mealtime ritual. Talking to local doctors and medical researchers, I learned that they ascribed several health benefits to the regular moderate intake of alcohol. Before we explore this area, "Let me make one thing perfectly clear," as President Nixon once said. I am reporting the medical data and research as it relates to the potential health benefits of alcohol. If you do not use alcohol I am *not* recommending that you start. As a board certified addiction specialist I recognize that alcohol has many negative consequences. However, the majority of scientific research indicates enough health benefits from moderate intake to justify endorsing such a pattern of usage for those who choose to partake.

Positive health effects of moderate alcohol intake include protection from the top 10 killer diseases and even an overall reduction in death rates compared to heavy drinkers or tee-totalers.

According to the *Mind-Body Health Newsletter (MBHN)*, "A host of studies indicate a reduction of mortality (death) from heart disease by about a third." Drinking two to six servings of alcohol per week reduces the risk of sudden death from heart attack in healthy men in one long-term study.

Moderate alcohol intake also reduced the risk of developing type-2 diabetes in women drinkers as compared to teetotalers, according to the authors of the Miami Community Health Study. These researchers attributed the reduced risk to alcohol's effect of increasing the body's sensitivity to insulin.

Pantry Prevention

Another study showed that one drink a day also protected against declining mental function, including Alzheimer's disease.

French scientists reported a 30% reduction in deaths from all causes for those who drank two or three glasses of wine a day.

For patients who have had a heart attack, their risk of dying is related to their intake of alcohol. Teetotalers had a 22% death rate compared to 13% for light drinkers. Moderate drinkers had the lowest death rate of 9%, according to Dr. Mukamal, a Harvard Medical School researcher.

While visiting a Swiss hospital in 1999, I noticed they served beer and wine in the cafeteria and coffee shop. This makes more sense than providing places to smoke, as many American hospitals do. Other benefits from alcohol included a 35% reduction in death from heart disease and an 18 to 24% reduction in cancer. A report in *FPN* (December 2000) noted that wine drinkers showed significantly less colon and rectal cancer compared to those who drank beer, liquor, or no alcohol at all. Dr. Carolyn Messina, author of the study, said this protective effect of wine is due to its action as an antioxidant.

The benefits of alcohol are not limited to those who drink wine. Beer drinkers, take heart! Your moderate drinking protects you from heart attacks by increasing levels of vitamin B-6, which in turn lowers the levels of homcysteine, a chemical in the bloodstream associated with an increase in heart disease. Beer may also be protective against cancer cells. Japanese investigators tested 24 beers from around the world including 17 lagers, four stouts, two ales, and a non-alcoholic brew. While most beers were found to inhibit cancer-causing chemicals, stouts were most effective. The non-alcoholic variety had no beneficial effect at all!

Once or twice a month my neighbor Perry and I relax in the evenings by sitting on his veranda as he sips his scotch and water and I down a low-alcohol beer. Part of the benefit of alcohol may be due to the relaxation and pleasure of slowing down and enjoying the company of a friend or neighbor (as we will see in the Positive Passions section).

Health Yourself

Two recent studies showed that wine drinkers have healthier habits than other drinkers. Those who drink mostly wine tend to have healthier diets and are less likely to smoke or be overweight compared to those who drink other forms of alcohol.

Strokes, or "brain attacks," are one of the leading causes of death and long-term disability and they come in two varieties: wet and dry. Ischemic or dry strokes are caused by a reduction or stoppage of blood flow in a certain part of the brain, while bleeding into the brain causes a hemorrhagic or wet stroke. Researchers found that adults consuming one or two drinks per day had 45% less risk of an ischemic stroke compared to non-drinkers. However, heavy drinkers (more than seven drinks a day) had three times the risk of an ischemic stroke compared to moderate or non-drinkers.

The ability of alcohol to prevent strokes may be due to its effect of reducing blood clots that often form blockages in the circulation to the brain, according to the results of the Physician's Health Study as reported in *FPN* (1999). Another possible explanation may be the mechanism by which alcohol raises the HDL ("good" cholesterol) that has a protective effect on the heart and circulation. The only other activity known to raise HDL is exercise, but a recent study showed alcohol raised HDL in women more than exercise did! Recently, when I was in Montana teaching PRO-vention at a nurses' convention, I spent an afternoon hiking and mountain climbing and afterwards rewarded myself with a couple of locally brewed beers at the pub at the base of the mountain. This combination of exercise and alcohol was the perfect prescription for raising my HDL, and it might work for you as well.

For patients who suffer a stroke, the future may hold a treatment based on the combined beneficial effects of coffee and alcohol. Stroke research expert Dr. James Grotta foresees the day when "a paramedic will scoop up a stroke patient and say, 'Here, have some coffee and a shot of bourbon.'"

Dr. Grotta, a Texas-based researcher, based his prediction on the results of his research on strokes in rats, which his colleagues dubbed "The Kahlua Project." The combination of two cups of coffee and one shot of whisky proved at least

Pantry Prevention

as effective in treating the damage of ischemic (dry) strokes as did more traditional medications. Dr. Grotta cautions that more research is needed before these results can be applied to humans, but I say the future is quite promising for an expanded role of alcohol in preventing and treating strokes.

When my diabetic friend Earl had his heart attack, he asked me if he would have to give up drinking his nightly beer. "Earl," I said, "the medical research says that compared to non-drinkers, you will lower your risk of having a repeat heart attack by 79% if you keep drinking a beer every day." Earl smiled and said he appreciated not having to give up another enjoyable aspect of his life because of his diabetes and heart disease. (I based this recommendation on a study in *JAMA* that was reported in the *AFP* in December, 1999.)

If you have already had a heart attack, alcohol may be part of your long-term recovery and protection. Men who had heart attacks and afterwards drank moderate alcohol had lower death rates than those men who did not drink alcohol. Those who drank two to six servings per week had the lowest death rates. Moderate drinking, defined as two to six drinks per week, reduced the risk of sudden death from a heart attack, according to another 12-year-long study. Having five or six drinks per week reduced the risk 79% while two to four drinks per week reduced the risk by 60%.

Researchers monitored a group of women for their drinking patterns and health status for over 20 years and found that those women who consumed one to three drinks per week gained the greatest health benefits. See the Illustration below for a breakdown of what one drink actually consists of.

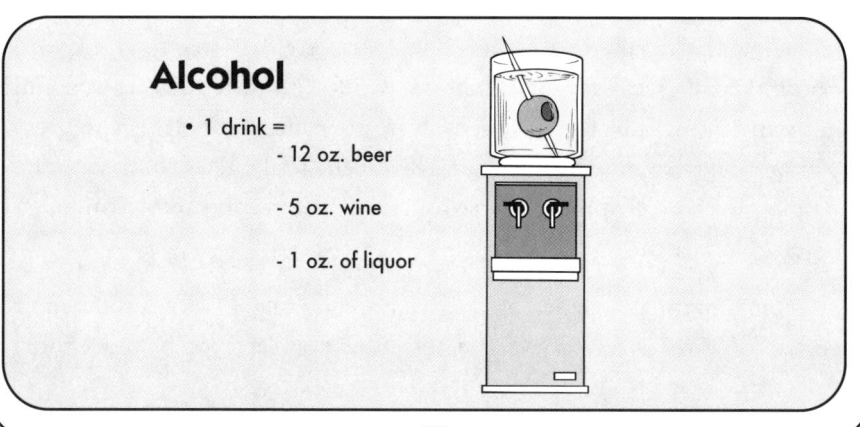

Alcohol
- 1 drink =
  - 12 oz. beer
  - 5 oz. wine
  - 1 oz. of liquor

Health Yourself

Avoiding congestive heart failure, a condition of excess fluid in the body caused by the heart's inability to pump efficiently, is another benefit of moderate alcohol intake according to a recent article in *JAMA*.

If you choose not to partake in alcohol, I am not suggesting you start now. However, for those who imbibe, I prescribe moderate intake in the appropriate setting for enjoyment, relaxation, social lubrication, and reducing the risk of several medical problems. Dr. R. Doll, writing in a 1997 issue of the *British Medical Journal*, summarized my recommendation on alcohol when he said, "Once we reach middle age, enjoying some small amount of alcohol (one to two drinks per day) reduces the risk of premature death."

Caution: alcohol can aggravate certain medical conditions such as high blood pressure and stomach ulcers and can impair your ability to drive or operate machinery. Remember, we define moderate drinking as two to three drinks per day for men and one to two per day for women. A serving of alcohol is 12 ounces of beer, four ounces of wine, or one ounce of hard liquor.

Tea Time

If alcohol is not your cup of tea, or even if it is, you may enjoy drinking tea and reaping its many health benefits. Tea drinking originated in the Orient nearly half a million years ago, according to Dr. Dennis McKenna's extensively researched article "Green Tea Monograph" (*Alternative Therapies*, May 2000). Ancient writings from around 780 A.D. indicate that Chinese herbalists used tea for medicinal purposes. Any way you look at it, tea drinkers in Asian countries have known for centuries that tea is useful in promoting weight loss as well as in treating ailments ranging from respiratory illness to digestive diseases. These beneficial effects along with the simple pleasure of sipping tea have made it the second most consumed beverage on earth.

Tea comes in three varieties: black, green, and oolong. Black tea is the most common commercial variety and the most popular type in the United

Pantry Prevention

States and is characterized by undergoing a chemical reaction shortly after the tea is picked. During the drying and curing, the process of fermentation occurs. This imparts the color of the tea and results in the chemical compounds that provide the many health benefits. Oolong teas are usually reddish or yellow and are only partially fermented, while green tea is unfermented and its chemical composition closely resembles the unprocessed leaves. Green tea contains more of the helpful compounds than black or oolong teas.

Green teas contain chemicals that fight cancer, reduce hardening of the arteries, and promote healthy bone growth to guard against osteoporosis. Black tea, the most common kind we drink in the United States, is the fermented version of green tea. Fermentation changes the chemical makeup of the tea, but black tea shares many of the healthy properties of green tea. In addition, black teas contain chemicals that reduce the build-up of plaque on your teeth and also help control bacteria in the mouth, which in return reduces the risks of cavities and gum disease. Experts have proposed that the bacteria that cause gum disease and tooth loss may contribute to the development of heart disease and hardening of the arteries.

A recent medical journal article reported that a group of 50 patients who drank four cups of tea a day for four weeks had improved circulation and better functioning blood vessels compared to non-tea drinkers.

A Boston area study found that drinking one cup of tea a day or more reduced the risk of heart attack by 44%, probably due to tea's ability to block the absorption of cholesterol.

Another group of researchers showed that green tea prevents tumor growth, and Chinese researchers noted significant mental improvement in Alzheimer's patients treated with tea supplements for one month.

Women in a weight loss study who took green tea supplement capsules lost twice as much weight compared to those who did not receive the supplements.

Health Yourself

Tea also contains chemicals that improve bone density and may help prevent osteoporosis and deadly fractures.

Researchers reporting in the *Journal of Nutrition* found that people who drank five 10-ounce servings of oolong tea for three days increased their energy output three percent more than those who drank plain water. That translates into burning an additional 67 calories a day, which over a year yields a six-and-a-half-pound weight loss. Comparing green tea extract to caffeine or a placebo, another group of researchers found that those who received green tea extract had a four percent advantage in energy expenditure (*American Journal of Clinical Nutrition*, reported in *Family Circle* magazine, October 2002).

Dr. McKenna also reports that in one study of 60 middle-aged obese women, the green tea group lost three times as much weight as the placebo group. Those receiving tea also had greater reductions in waist size and had a significant improvement in their lipid profiles.

Green tea also helps prevent cancer. Researchers in one Japanese study found that a minimum of three cups per day led to a decreased incidence of all cancers. Other studies found tea reduced the risk for stomach cancer and pancreatic and colorectal cancer, and it is even associated with a decreased risk of recurrence for stage I and II breast cancers.

Medical experts caution that tea alone cannot prevent heart disease, but it can be part of an overall healthy lifestyle.

Researchers at the University of Arizona Cancer Center recommend squeezing a little lemon into your tea to reduce the chance of skin cancer. Regularly drinking tea and eating citrus peel were linked to a 70% reduction in skin cancer. Due to their increased dilution, iced drinks are less effective than hot ones.

Caution: tea contains caffeine, just like coffee and sodas, which acts as a diuretic and can lead to dehydration and loss of fluids. Nutritionists recommend drinking an *extra* glass of water for each caffeinated beverage you drink.

Pantry Prevention

Advice from *The Tea Companion, a Connoisseur's Guide* (John Wiley and Sons) by Jane Pettigrew and David Prebenna outlines the characteristics of each type of tea and offers tips on proper brewing techniques (*Family Circle,* October 2002): "…Start with good quality tea leaves (tea bags may be used). Fill a kettle with cold water and bring to a boil. Put the leaves in the bottom of a separate pot or in an infuser inside the pot (one teaspoon tea leaves per cup of water). Pour the boiled water onto the leaves. Put the lid on the pot and let brew for several minutes. To avoid the tea steeping too long and developing a bitter taste, decant the brewed tea into a second warmed pot, separating the liquid from the leaves. (If using an infuser or tea bags, there's no need to pour the tea into a second pot.) Remove the infuser or bag once the tea has reached its desired strength."

If you're unsure of what type of tea to try, the following guidelines from *The Tea Companion* might help:

Oolong: has a light, peachy, mild taste and pairs well with light or spicy foods or is good after a meal.

Green: is aromatic and refreshing and is best served with a snack or after dinner.

Darjeeling: has a pronounced aroma and serves as an afternoon tea.

Ceylon: is a rich blend with a brisk flavor and is often served with breakfast

Keemun: is a Chinese black tea with a scented aroma and is best used after dinner.

Earl Grey: is a blended tea with a refreshing citrus flavor best for accompanying cheeses, fish, or meat.

Jasmine: is the result of infusing black, green, or oolong tea with the scent of jasmine flowers; it pairs well with spicy foods, meat, and poultry.

"Choosing tea as often as you can as your beverage is more important than which kind of tea you choose," says Dr. Jeffrey Blumberg, professor of nutrition at Tufts University in Boston. Dr. Blumberg notes that bottled iced teas have nearly undetectable levels of beneficial chemicals because they diminish rapidly with exposure to light and oxygen. Homemade iced tea is slightly better than the bottled version but not nearly as concentrated as the hot tea.

Health Yourself

All Juiced Up

Adding the right kinds of juice to your diet can be good for you, too.

Cranberry Juice. Long recognized as a folk remedy or preventive for bladder infections, the benefits of cranberry juice have now been confirmed by research. Studies show that chemicals in the juice block the ability of bacteria to stick to the bladder wall and cause infection. Women who drank a concentrate of cranberry-lingonberry juice daily (50 cc, a little less than two ounces) had only half as many repeat infections as those who did not drink the juice (*British Medical Journal* [*BMJ*], September 2001).

Women who drank 10 ounces of cranberry juice daily had reduced infection rates over six months.

Tomato Juice. The more concentrated and processed forms of tomatoes provide a more enriched source of the beneficial chemicals known as lycopenes compared to the fresh version of tomatoes. Lycopenes help protect men against prostate cancer and also lower the risk of other cancers as well.

Orange Juice. According to a report from the American Heart Association (*FPN*, 2000), three glasses of orange juice daily may help prevent hardening of the arteries. This regimen of three glasses a day for four weeks produced a 21% increase in "good" cholesterol (HDL), which is known to have a protective effect on the arteries and the heart.

Besides protecting the heart, OJ can also aid in fertility. When sperm stick to each other the odds of impregnation are reduced. Men who consumed 500 milligrams of vitamin C twice a day had a nearly 50% decrease in the number of sperm sticking together.

Grape Juice. A 1999 report in *Medical Tribune* (*MT*) showed that purple grapes contain chemicals that protect circulation and the heart. Dr. John Folts, a researcher from Wisconsin, says chemicals called flavinoids are the key ingredient in the protective effect of grapes. Found not only in grape juice and red wines but also in fruits, vegetables, nuts, and seeds, flavinoids

Pantry Prevention

act as natural blood thinners. Dr. Folts says this helps explain the "French Paradox": people in France eat four times as much saturated fat as Americans but have one-third the risk of heart disease.

White wine contains only one-seventh the flavinoids of red wines.

Another research project in Wisconsin found that heart patients who consumed a liter of ordinary grape juice daily improved the function of their blood vessels and reduced their risk of another heart attack.

Cherry Juice. Rheumatologist Dr. James Mckoy advises that drinking tart cherry juice mixed with water three times a day may be beneficial for some patients with arthritis. Dr. Mckoy cautions that the beneficial effects of cherry juice have not yet been proven by research, but he reasons that chemicals in cherries have anti-inflammatory properties similar to medications used to treat arthritis (*WB*, October 2002).

Pomegranate Juice. Israeli scientists found that pomegranate juice can help protect the heart by preventing the development of plaque in the arteries and by reducing the damaging effects of "bad" cholesterol (LDL) (*American Journal of Clinical Nutrition*, May 2000). Drinking a half-cup of pomegranate juice daily may give you more heart protection than wine. Pomegranate juice had five times the amount of polyphenols, the heart healthy chemicals that lowered "bad" cholesterol and reduced heart disease risk by 44%.

Food and Nutrition – The Final Word

Almost everyone has seen or heard of the American Heart Association's nutritional guideline known as the "Food Pyramid," but very few of us follow its recommendations. Is it because it was designed by the food pharaohs?

We think of food and nutrition as sources of enjoyment and energy, but what we eat can also have positive health benefits as well. Healthy dietary habits are the foundation of a healthy lifestyle and both are a matter of choice. Luckily, some of the confusion in the dietary guidelines has

Health Yourself

disappeared with the release of the Unified Dietary Guidelines developed jointly by the American Heart Association, the American Cancer Society, the American Dietetic Association, the American Academy of Pediatrics, and the National Institutes of Health. All of these organizations endorse the following basic recommendations:

1. Eat five to six servings of fruits and vegetables daily.
2. Eat six or more servings of grain-based foods daily.
3. Limit total fat intake to less than 30% of total daily calories.
4. Eat a variety of foods mainly from plant sources.
5. Limit polyunsaturated fats to less than 10% of your total daily calories.
6. Limit monosaturated fats to less than 15% of your total daily calories.
7. Eat at least half your calories from complex carbohydrates.
8. Limit simple carbohydrates such as table sugar.

Now that you know more about the abundance of healthy and enjoyable foods, you can make better and wiser choices that can improve your health profile and give you a longer and higher quality life.

The Kitchen Medicine Cabinet

Herbal and plant substances, also a part of the pantry, have been shown to have medicinal and positive health effects, though they are not necessarily enjoyable in the same way as candy or alcohol. One goal of PRO-vention is to teach you how to be your own "doctor" in certain situations. Using herbal and plant-based products can be a safe and effective way for you to treat minor illnesses yourself and also provide some preventive measures as well.

This is not meant to be an exhaustive and complete resource for the subject of herbal remedies, sometimes referred to as "complementary," "alternative," or "integrative" medicine. I refer you to the website for resources and links that go into much more detail on these topics. Again, I

Pantry Prevention

remind you that this is not intended to be specific individual medical advice but a broad general explanation.

Feverfew. A common garden flower known as "summer daisy," feverfew has long been used as a folk remedy for arthritis, fever, and headaches. Once strictly a European plant, feverfew is now grown in the U.S. and Canada and has yellow leaves and flowers when in bloom from July to October. Feverfew leaves are dried and then used in teas or extracts for the treatment of asthma, dental pain, psoriasis, fever, and stomach pain. Recent research shows feverfew to also be a promising treatment for migraine headaches. While feverfew doesn't help much after the headaches start, it is useful in preventing the onset of migraines and reducing the associated symptoms of nausea and vomiting.

According to experts, the best source of feverfew is the homegrown variety. Two to three fresh leaves daily taken as supplements with your regular meals is the recommended dose. Feverfew is also available in capsule, liquid, and tablet forms.

Caution: Feverfew may interact with aspirin and other anti-inflammatory drugs such as ibuprofen and other arthritis drugs. Consult with your physician or pharmacist before taking feverfew if you are taking any of these types of drugs. Children and pregnant or nursing women should not take feverfew.

Chamomile. "True" chamomile refers to the variety known as Hungarian or German, which is different from another form called Roman or English. Taking 400 to 1,600 milligrams daily as a pill or drinking chamomile tea can have a calming effect, reduce anxiety, and induce sleep. Chamomile is also useful as a remedy for stomach conditions such as indigestion, heartburn, excessive gas, and can be used as mouthwash for infected and inflamed gums and sore throats. Other possible benefits include treatment of various skin disorders, menstrual pain, and eye irritation.

Caution: people with severe allergy to ragweed may also have a similar reaction to chamomile. If you take large doses of chamomile to treat insomnia, avoid driving or operating machinery. If you are taking prescription medications to treat depression, chamomile may reduce their effectiveness.

Evening Primrose. This peppery flavored herb grows wild in North America and Europe. Supplements containing this herb may be useful in treating symptoms of PMS and menopause. Doses of two to eight grams daily in the form of capsules and gel caps may also relieve symptoms of rheumatoid arthritis, psoriasis, and diabetic nerve damage.

Caution: Patients with schizophrenia, seizures, or on medications for psychosis should avoid evening primrose.

Ginseng. Oriental healers have used the power of ginseng for over two millennia as an aphrodisiac and to treat liver diseases, diabetes, depression, and decreased mental function. Ginseng grown in the wild in Oriental countries is usually processed by drying or curing, whereas the American form of ginseng undergoes less processing and is not considered as valuable or effective.

Daily intake of 200 to 600 milligrams enhances mental and physical activity, increases energy, decreases stress, improves immune function, and is useful for those patients receiving radiation or chemotherapy.

Ginseng is sold as capsules, powder, extract, and teabags.

Caution: Do not take ginseng if you have kidney failure or are taking the heart drug digitalis. Long-term use is not advised for patients with high blood pressure.

Be especially careful with ginseng if you are taking medications for diabetes. Use ginseng cautiously if you are taking blood thinners. Do not use ginseng if you are pregnant or have an acute infection.

Echinacea. Some people use this herb, available as a juice, powder, or tea, to treat burns, skin inflammation, respiratory infections, and urinary tract infections. Claims that echinacea can cure the common cold have not been scientifically proven, though some evidence suggests that it may be useful for reducing symptoms during the early stages of a respiratory infection.

Caution: Echinacea should not be used more than eight weeks at a time. Those sensitive to ragweed may experience allergic reactions to echinacea. Pregnancy and breastfeeding are reasons to avoid echinacea altogether.

Saw Palmetto. The brownish-black fruit from this small scrubby palm tree (American dwarf palm) that grows in the southeastern U.S. has been used for centuries to treat men's urinary problems. Working the same way in the body as many prescription drugs for prostate trouble, saw palmetto relieves

Pantry Prevention

the symptoms of mild to moderate prostate enlargement such as hesitant urination and irritable bladder. The average dose is 160 milligrams twice a day. Saw Palmetto is available over the counter in supermarkets, drug stores, and health food stores.

Caution: Saw palmetto may aggravate high blood pressure.

Melatonin. Melatonin is not a true herb but a hormone produced in the pineal gland, a tiny area at the base of the brain. Melatonin has a reputation for regulating sleep cycles and treating jet lag and my doctor friend Tony said it worked very well on his 17-hour flight to Australia. Side effects include headache, itching, mental cloudiness, and an increased heart rate.

Caution: Patients who have a history of stroke, depression, or other neurological disorders are not candidates for melatonin.

St. John's Wort. Derived from a flower that produces red oil, legend has it that this plant first grew out of the blood of John the Baptist following his decapitation. Native to Europe and Asia, early colonists brought St. John's Wort (Hypericum) to the American colonies.

Used as a treatment for mild to moderate depression, nervousness, and anxiety, 200 to 300 milligrams up to three times a day is the recommended dosage. The problem with St. John's Wort along with other over-the-counter herbals is that there is no standardization between the various brands. One brand may be twice as potent as another brand offering the same dosage in milligrams.

Caution: Side effects may include fatigue and stomach upset. Light-skinned patients may have increased sensitivity to sunlight. Never take this while taking prescription antidepressants. Always tell your doctor if you are taking St. John's Wort or any other herbal medication.

Gingko Biloba. Made from extracts of the maidenhair or kew tree, gingko has been around for thousands of years as an Oriental curative and is a popular prescription drug in Europe.

Gingko may improve circulation and increase mental function in Alzheimer's patients and has also proved beneficial in treating vertigo, headaches, and ringing of the ears. It has antioxidant properties that reduce inflammation and has no known toxic effects and few side effects.

Health Yourself

However, these include stomach upset, headache, and skin irritation.

Valerian Root. Europeans have long used valerian as a sedative and for treatment of muscular spasms. It is also a mild tranquilizer used to treat insomnia and symptoms of nervousness during PMS and menopause.

Caution: Valerian root can worsen drowsiness caused by other medications and alcohol.

Garlic. Eating garlic may increase your chances of living to be 100 years old. Health experts found a region in China that has seven times as many 100-year-olds as other Chinese regions. Most of these centenarians live in the garlic-producing region of the province and include large amounts of garlic in their diets.

Garlic contains vitamins, amino acids, and proteins and can fight against more than 100 types of harmful bacteria, as well as prevent flu and other diseases, according to an article in the May 2001 issue of *Healthworld Online*.

In short, while herbal supplements can help alleviate certain health problems, caution is in order. Dr. Michael Cirigliano at the University of Pennsylvania Medical School wrote the following "12 Commandments" of safely using herbals for doctors in a recent medical journal. I have adapted them so they are applicable to you, the patients:

The 12 commandments of using herbal medications

1. Always tell your doctor or health care provider if you are using any herbal therapies or dietary supplements.

2. "Natural" or "herbal" doesn't necessarily mean safe.

3. Herbal medications can react with regular prescription medications, so avoid combining the two.

4. Beware the lack of standardization, which may result in wide variability in content between brands.

Pantry Prevention

5. Lack of quality control and regulation may result in contamination during the manufacturing process, leading to potential misidentification of plant species.

6. Avoid herbal treatments if you are pregnant or contemplating pregnancy or if you are breastfeeding.

7. Don't take more than the recommended dosage. More is not always better!

8. Limit usage to a few weeks due to lack of studies proving long-term safety.

9. Avoid using herbal medications with known toxic effects.

10. Infants, children, and the elderly should not use herbal treatments without professional advice.

11. Always discuss your condition and potential proven treatment options with your health care provider before starting herbal therapy.

12. Always advise your doctor if you experience any negative side effects so they can be documented in your medical record.

Vitamins, additives, and supplements commonly found in the kitchen medicine cabinet can also help keep us healthy. "10 years from now, we'll prevent strokes by giving patients a multivitamin," says Dr. J. D. Spence, director of the Stroke Prevention Program in London. His research showed that a multivitamin supplement of folic acid, B vitamins, and E vitamins slowed the rate of blockage in the blood vessels that supply the brain. Higher levels of vitamin C were also associated with reduced plaques, the blockages in the circulation that lead to strokes. Let's take a brief look at some of the common vitamins we can use to health ourselves!

Vitamin C. Essential to the formation of collagen, the "glue" that holds bones and body tissues together, many scientific studies show vitamin C to have potential effects against cancer, heart disease, and cataracts. Research also indicates that 250 to 500 milligrams of vitamin C helps reduce the duration and severity of common cold symptoms or to prevent infection altogether. Researchers at the University of Alabama found that larger-than-usual doses of vitamin C may prevent illness by reducing the levels of stress hormones in the body. These animal studies may apply to humans as well.

Health Yourself

Combining vitamin C and vitamin E proved to slow down the process of hardening of the arteries, especially in smokers.

New research suggests vitamin C may be beneficial for those patients whose asthma symptoms are triggered by exercise. Two grams of vitamin C one hour before exercise on a treadmill improved symptoms of asthma for 50% of patients.

Vitamin E. This powerful antioxidant is found in nuts, vegetable oils, and seeds and may help prevent cancer, heart disease, and cataracts. Recent studies indicate that it may also be effective in preventing Alzheimer's disease. Supplements of 400 to 1,000 milligrams daily supply the required amount of vitamin E.

Vitamin D. Your body needs vitamin D to absorb and use calcium, an important part of bone health. Sources include natural sunlight, fortified milk, and multivitamin supplements.

Vitamin K. Usually noted for its effect on blood clotting, vitamin K promotes the production of three bone proteins necessary for strength. Eating broccoli and leafy greens can produce high levels of vitamin K, which in turn can help prevent hip fractures.

Folic Acid. This B vitamin prevents certain birth defects and now is known to reduce the risk of heart disease. Researchers studied over 80,000 women and found that those with the most folate in their diet had a 47% reduction in their risk for heart disease. Cancer prevention is also a possibility for this vitamin, which occurs naturally in fruits, vegetables, fortified grains, and cereals. Experts recommend supplements of 400 micrograms per day in addition to natural sources.

Cold breakfast cereal, spinach, tuna, and milk are all excellent sources of folic acid.

Final Pantry Prevention Tips

Let's finish up this first section with some tips designed to make you and the ones you love happier and healthier.

Pantry Prevention

Never Too Young

Giving infants multivitamin supplements resulted in reduced rates of a disease process that leads to diabetes. The liquid vitamin supplement contained a full spectrum of vitamins but researchers credit vitamin E and its antioxidant effect for most of the protective properties.

Bone Up on Bone Health

Besides vitamins, there are other chemicals that are important to your health. One of the most important is calcium. Experts agree that calcium is one of the most important minerals in the body since it is the primary ingredient in your bones. Imagine yourself without any bones to keep your body straight! But bones are more than just a support system for your muscles and do far more than keep you upright. As hard as concrete on the outside, bones are soft and spongy on the inside and are constantly involved in the body's chemical reactions. Unlike the dry dead bones you see on Halloween skeletons, your bones are living tissues that are always undergoing changes and remodeling under the influence of hormones, testosterone in men and estrogen in women. Calcium is deposited in the bones and then released into the circulation for the body to use in its chemical reactions. When the amount of calcium leaving the bones exceeds the amount deposited, bones are thinned out and weakened, a condition known as osteoporosis.

Taking calcium supplements can prevent this condition from developing. When you take calcium into your body, either from foods or supplements, it does not go directly to your bones. Every chemical reaction in your body requires calcium, and if you have an adequate level in your bloodstream, your body doesn't have to "borrow" calcium from your bones. Taking extra calcium allows your bones to hang on to their calcium and they do not become washed out and weakened.

Women, especially post-menopausal Caucasian ones, are more likely to develop osteoporosis than men, and there are certain other conditions that increase the risk of developing weaker bones. Smoking, taking thyroid

Health Yourself

supplements, blood thinners, or steroid medications, being thin, and physical inactivity all increase your risk for osteoporosis. These weak bones don't make you feel bad or sick, but they increase the risk of hip fractures and other broken bones. The death rates from these fractures are higher than for some types of cancer.

So, how can you enjoy yourself while protecting yourself from developing osteoporosis? Low-fat dairy products such as skim milk and low-fat yogurt can supply some of your calcium requirements, but most experts recommend additional supplements. Taking pills isn't much fun, but there are caramel candy-like squares available that contain adequate calcium and few calories.

Calcium is not only necessary for bone health, it is also a key factor in many of the body's functions and chemical reactions. Eating foods rich in calcium and taking supplements protects your bones by providing an adequate level of the mineral in your bloodstream.

Regular intake of calcium can also lower blood pressure and reduces the risk of breast and colon cancer. Recent studies show that dietary calcium lowers both the top and bottom blood pressure numbers. Dairy food sources of calcium drop the blood pressure twice as low as calcium supplements. Blood vessels are rich in calcium receptors, which control the muscle tone of the blood vessels. Calcium lowers blood pressure by providing adequate calcium supplies for the vessels to function properly at lower pressures.

Diets high in fats and low in calcium may be one reason that colon cancer has become the second leading cancer killer right behind lung cancer. Researchers suspect that calcium's protective effect comes from its ability to bind fats and bile acids in the colon and help the body get rid of those cancer-causing chemicals.

Calcium intake can also protect you from forming kidney stones. For years doctors advised people with stones to avoid calcium, the main ingredient in most stones. We now know this was bad advice. Chemicals in the urine called oxylates form kidney stones. Contrary to popular belief, calcium lowers the risk of forming kidney stones by binding up the oxylates and flushing them out of the body.

Pantry Prevention

Calcium is also beneficial in regulating the heartbeat and helping blood form healing clots. It also helps muscles grow and function and helps nerves transmit messages from one part of the body to another. Calcium helps the body use iron, regulates the passage of nutrients in and out of body cells, and activates other chemicals that help food work in the body.

Calcium supplements, which improve bone health, may also protect women from the symptoms of PMS such as bloating, breast tenderness, headaches, and mood disorders.

Women aren't the only ones who need calcium. Men are susceptible to brittle bones, too, and teenagers, especially girls, should also take calcium regularly as their growing bones are more prone to breaking. The recommended dose for men and pre-menopausal women is one gram daily, but after menopause, women need at least one and a half grams per day. Children ages six through adolescence also benefit from calcium, as it builds up their bone mass and lessens their chances for osteoporosis later in life. The dose for teens is one to one and a half grams per day. See the following chart for a rundown on recommended doses.

Recommended calcium intake
The DASH eating plan below is based on a 2,000 calorie a day diet.

Group	Amount (mg/d)
Adolescents and young adults	1200-1500
Adults aged 25-50 years	1000
Pregnant and nursing women	1200-1500
Postmenopausal women	1000-1500

Source: US Preventive Services Task Force. Guide to clinical preventive services. 2nd ed. Baltimore, Md: Williams & Wilkins. 1995.

Although there are many forms of calcium available, all calcium supplements are not the same. Tums, usually sold as antacid tablets, contains calcium car-

Health Yourself

bonate, an inexpensive form of calcium. Researchers say calcium carbonate is "a good source of calcium" in terms of quantity, but it is poorly absorbed.

Calcium citrate is a supplement available as Citracal that provides two and a half times as much calcium to the bloodstream as calcium carbonate.

While calcium is important to bone health, other factors such as hormones and physical activity come into play as well. Combining regular exercise with a calcium-rich diet can increase sports performance and reduce the risk of fractures. Walking or some other form of physical activity can improve the overall health of your bones. Working in the yard at least once a week can have the same protective effect against osteoporosis as weight training, according to University of Arkansas researchers who studied a group of 3,000 women. Dr. Lori Turner noted that "Pushing a mower and digging in flowerbeds involves upper-and lower-body weight-bearing motion which increases bone density. Plus, just being outside will help build strong bones. Sunshine encourages your body to produce vitamin D, which boosts calcium absorption."

Three eight-ounce glasses of milk each day (skim milk has zero fat calories) helps bone health and provides the protein necessary for repairing strained muscles after a workout. See the table below for the top five food sources of calcium:

The top five food sources of calcium

(adapted from *Managing Menopause Magazine*, Fall 2002)

Yogurt, plain, low-fat (1 cup, 8 ounces)	415 mg.
Yogurt, fruit, low-fat (1 cup)	314 mg.
Skim milk (1 cup)	302 mg.
Swiss cheese (1 ounce)	272 mg.
Cheddar cheese (1 ounce)	204 mg.

Pantry Prevention

Magnesium, found in green vegetables, beans, and nuts, is equally as important as calcium in bone health. Potassium, found in bananas and oranges, helps keep the calcium inside the bones and also reduces blood pressure and thus lowers the risk of strokes and heart attack. Potassium is the main ingredient in many "salt substitutes" used to spice up meals. Always check with your doctor before using a salt substitute or any other form of potassium.

Trace minerals such as copper, manganese, and zinc are valuable in maintaining collagen, sometimes called connective tissue, the "glue" that holds your body tissues together. Eating nuts, shellfish, beans, and chocolate will supply your body with copper. Eating pennies won't help, since they contain very little if any copper. Manganese sources include whole grains, nuts, berries, beans, shellfish, and tea. Zinc is found in meat, seafood, and liver.

Aspirin

Aspirin can also play a role in your health. Back in the 1960s there was a joke going around that aspirin could be used as a birth control pill if girls held it between their knees. While aspirin is not a very effective contraceptive, it has many positive health benefits for those who can tolerate it.

Small doses of aspirin (81 to 325 milligrams) can protect against heart disease, stroke, and colon cancer. For women, aspirin may reduce the odds of developing ovarian cancer by up to 40%. Men aren't left out completely, either. One study by the National Institute on Aging showed that taking aspirin regularly may reduce the risk of prostate cancer by 15 to 24%. The American Diabetic Association found that 98% of diabetics are candidates for aspirin but only 20% are taking the drug, which protects those at a higher risk for heart disease.

A study in *JAMA* reported, "Regular aspirin use can markedly reduce heart disease-related deaths across the board." Experts recommend "routine use of aspirin in patients with, or at risk for, cardiovascular disease." Once used mainly as a pain killer, aspirin is now known to not only prevent heart disease, but also to reduce the death rate from all causes.

Health Yourself

Everyone over age 50 with one or more risk factors for heart disease (see the chart below) should take aspirin daily unless they have an allergy to aspirin or some other reason to avoid aspirin.

Cardiac risk factors

1. Male gender
2. Increasing age
3. Family history of heart disease
4. Diabetes
5. Elevated cholesterol
6. High blood pressure
7. Sedentary lifestyle
8. Obesity
9. Job dissatisfaction
10. Smoking and tobacco use

My Uncle Doo-Dad says his doctor told him the aspirin would work even better if he put it in his pocket and took it for a three-mile walk before he swallowed it.

Check with your doctor or health care provider to determine if aspirin may be good for you.

Glucosamine and Chondroitin Sulfate

These over-the-counter supplements may be moderately effective in relieving the pain and immobility of osteoarthritis. While some studies showed these compounds provided effective symptom relief in patients with osteoarthritis of the hips and knees, experts say further research is needed to confirm these benefits.

Pantry Prevention

The recommended dosage of Glucosamine is 1,500 milligrams per day. For Chondroitin, the dosage is 1,200 milligrams per day.

Caution: Those with shellfish allergies should avoid Glucosamine since it is derived from shellfish that can set off serious allergic reactions. Animal studies showed that Glucosamine may interfere with insulin production and thus may pose some danger for diabetics.

Gel Your Knees

A gelatin-based dietary supplement improved knee function during walking, jogging, and other activities that stress these joints. The study showed that patients on the gel showed improvement in strength and work performance compared to those who received a placebo (inactive sugar pill).

Shake off the Salt

A salt-filled diet can lead to high blood pressure as well as other negative health consequences such as hardening of the arteries, which can cause a stroke. According to an article in the British medical journal *Lancet*, asthmatics may have fewer symptoms and less need for medication as a result of a lower salt intake. Other health conditions that may improve with salt reduction include fluid retention, abnormal enlargement of the heart, and osteoporosis. Reducing your intake of salt by half every day can yield some of these health benefits. Add spice by using herbal seasonings instead of regular salt.

Ditch the Diet

Recent surveys found that over half of adult Americans are overweight (mostly the bottom half) and childhood obesity has doubled in the past 20 years. Fat is more than just unsightly. A recent survey in *Business and Health* reported that "Obesity is worse for your health than smoking and drinking." Overweight people have almost twice as many chronic illnesses compared to

Health Yourself

their normal weight counterparts and have more health problems than smokers, drinkers, and those living in poverty.

Weight loss is a complex issue involving genetic, environmental, and behavioral issues and I cannot address the topic in great detail here, but I can offer a few nuggets of practical advice. If you are concerned about your weight and want some medical advice, don't wait for your doctor to bring up the subject. Speak up for yourself. A recent study illuminated the fact that fewer than 50% of doctors brought up the subject of obesity and weight loss with patients who were obviously overweight or suffering from weight-related conditions.

Remember, too, that "going on a diet" is one of the worst things you can do to lose weight. There are many weight loss "gurus" with a wide variety of diets they claim will help you lose weight, and these diets range from being just plain silly to being downright dangerous.

What's more, food restrictions, the cornerstone of dieting, appear to cause rebound weight gain, lowered self-esteem, and other psychological problems. People on restrictive diets tend to overindulge and binge once the restrictions are lifted. Food deprivation and restriction cause overactive emotions, depression, thinking difficulties, and excessive worry over food and weight. With all these increased worries, you are more likely to eat more and gain more weight! Instead of denying yourself the enjoyment of foods, focus on the wide variety of foods you can have in your eating plan and remember that moderation is the key to success in reaching and maintaining a healthier weight. Using the food pyramid approach as pictured on the following page may be helpful in making better choices.

Pantry Prevention

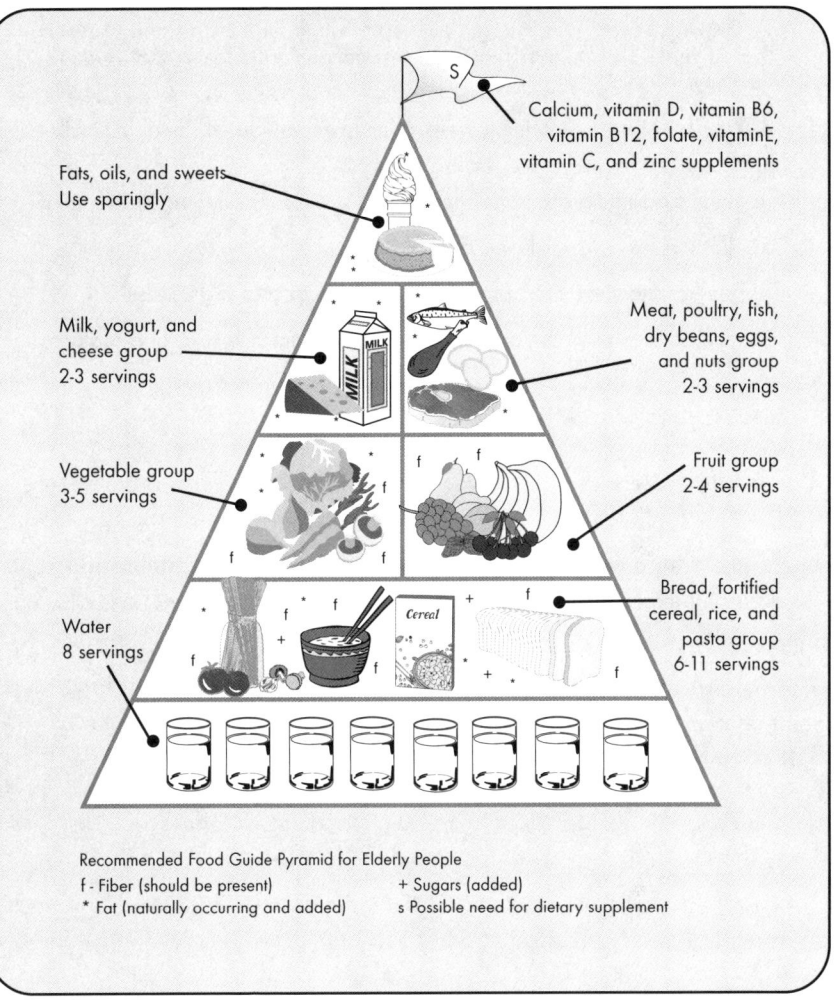

Recommended Food Guide Pyramid for Elderly People
f - Fiber (should be present)   + Sugars (added)
* Fat (naturally occurring and added)   s Possible need for dietary supplement

I prefer to heed the advice of those experts who recommend we eat *more* and not less. There is a wealth of scientific evidence to support the idea of "grazing" as the best way to eat. Six to 10 "mini-meals" has several advantages over the usual habit of "three squares a day" that most of us follow. An author summarized the findings from several research studies in *Running and Fitness News* and found grazing to have the following beneficial effects:

1. Grazing keeps your metabolism at an even rate and prevents wide swings caused by long periods of not eating.

Health Yourself

2. Grazing keeps your energy level up throughout the day and prevents those "peaks and valleys" that interfere with performance, mood, and productivity.

3. Your body uses proteins more efficiently when you eat them in smaller doses.

4. Small meals increase your energy level without making you feel too full.

5. Nibblers have lower levels of cholesterol.

6. Healthy snacking can help you eat more fruits and vegetables.

7. Eating after exercising promotes recovery of tired muscles and replaces lost energy stores.

The key to understanding weight loss is to think of your body's energy as *money*. The food you take in is a deposit of calories, and the calories you burn off through activity and exercise are the same as spending money. Just like your checkbook, if you deposit more than you spend, your balance increases. If you're like most of us, you know that if you spend more than you deposit, your balance decreases. So, gaining weight is nothing more than an energy imbalance where we take in more calories than we use up and the excess is stored as fat.

The checkbook analogy is such a good one that Dr. John Foreyt uses it in his weight loss clinic at Baylor Medical School. Dr. Foreyt says that patients who keep a food diary and record their deposits (food intake) and withdrawals (calories burned in physical activity) have a much higher success rate in weight loss than those who do not keep such a record.

Interestingly, vegetarians tend to maintain their weight loss dietary modifications for longer than a year compared to the rest of us, who average about three months. According to a University of Pittsburgh survey, the most common reasons for ditching weight loss diets are "I'm not losing any weight" and "I'm bored." If you follow the lead of the vegetarians and substitute interesting healthy foods for meat, you may overcome both excuses.

According to the February 2000 issue of *AM*, there are four habits of highly successful dieters:

Pantry Prevention

1. They "avoid the quick fix" by developing a long-term food plan that they always follow.

2. They choose foods they like rather than low-calorie or low-fat foods that don't taste good.

3. They practice portion control. They eat their favorite foods – just not quite so much of them. They resist the temptation to "super-size."

4. They plan for slip-ups. When they overindulge, as we all do, they don't try to make up for it by starving or fasting.

As a bonus, tip, try browsing the Internet along with the fridge. Patients who use interactive web sites as part of their weight loss program are more successful than those who use other learning materials. See the resource section for a listing of recommended websites. Also, visit www.healthyourselves.com for frequent updates.

Australian researchers also have a few tips for those trying to get the maximum sensation of fullness from the fewest calories (*UCBWL*, May 1996):

- Potatoes rank as the most filling food, seven times more filling than the last place croissant.
- Bread made from whole grains is 50% more filling than white bread.
- Snacks high in fat and sugar such as cakes, cookies, and doughnuts are among the least filling.
- Apples and oranges beat bananas.
- Fish is more filling per calorie than chicken or beef.
- Popcorn is twice as filling as a candy bar or peanuts.

Success in losing weight is measured by more than looking at the scales. You may be dissatisfied with losing only 10 to 15% of your body weight, but this small amount of loss can have many health benefits. Also, researchers tell us it is better to be a little overweight and physically fit than to be normal weight and unfit. Success is also defined by improvement in your overall energy level and sense of well-being.

Odd as it may sound, getting a little more sleep may help you lose weight. When we don't get enough sleep, our bodies produce less growth hormone, which in turn decreases lean muscles and increases fat. As we age, we sleep less and thus reduce our levels of growth hormone, a substance that breaks down fats and acts to reduce and redistribute body fat. More detailed research is needed to establish a direct link between sleep and weight gain, but improving your sleep patterns can have a positive effect on many other aspects of your life.

Taking care of yourself after you eat is important, too. No matter how healthy your food is, it can cause health problems if it stays around your teeth and gums too long. Researchers did dental check-ups on 44,000 men for eight years and found that those with fewer than 25 teeth had almost a 50% increase in their risk of stroke. Experts suspect that the bacteria in the mouth that cause gum disease and tooth loss play a role in causing heart disease and hardening of the arteries.

Regular brushing and flossing are cheap insurance against these killer diseases and may help in preventing weight loss due to after-dinner snacking. Brushing, flossing, and using a bacteria-fighting mouthwash *immediately* after eating distorts flavors and may also discourage snacking, a source of calories with little nutritional benefit.

Conclusion

So, now we know that when we put food, beverages, herbs, vitamins, and supplements in our mouths we help lower our risk of developing the conditions that most commonly cause people to die young. Foods are also a source of fuel and energy that we need in order to perform our routine activities of daily function and living as well as the enjoyable activities that I refer to as "Pleasurable Pursuits," the next step in learning how to health yourself.

Section Two

> *I seek the utmost pleasure and the least pain.*
>
> Plautus

How we spend our free time can have either a positive or a negative effect on our physical and mental health. A 1997 survey asked how we spend our leisure time, and the results showed that watching television was the favorite leisure activity for relaxation. Sixty eight percent of people chose the tube, compared to only 55% in 1993. Listening to music came in a close second at 67%, followed by sleeping, the favorite activity of 54%. Drinking alcohol came in last as the preferred leisure time activity for 24% compared to 18% in 1993.

Unfortunately, watching television confers very little in the way of health benefits as it is a passive activity that requires minimal intellectual or physical participation on the part of the observer. Television watchers subject themselves to a "triple whammy" of negative health consequences. First, watching television requires no physical activity and burns only a few calories per hour. Second, most programming is supported by advertisers whose products generally are not health oriented. Third, most television viewers are sprawled out in their recliners surrounded by high fat, high calorie junk snacks. Being glued to the tube also takes us away from interacting with others. Ann Landers, the late advice columnist, said, "Watching television proves that we would rather watch anything else than watch each other."

PLEASURABLE PURSUITS

Health Yourself

Other popular activities such as listening to music, sleeping, and drinking alcohol can all be part of a healthy lifestyle, but can also be damaging and unhealthy when pursued as a means to escape from the challenges of everyday life.

We are the sum of our choices in all areas of our lives. Our choices can lead us to lives of energy and fulfillment or to a lifetime of illness, disease, and negative feelings. In this section we will explore some choices for how you spend your free time that can be enjoyable and also improve your physical and mental health. I refer to these as "Pleasurable Pursuits," and I hope you learn something new to help you make better choices to replace channel surfing as your favorite activity.

Exercise – The Magic Pill

My first recommendation would be for you to graduate from being a couch potato to becoming a "hot potato," one that works up a little sweat and an increased heart rate from engaging in physical activity. Turning off the tube and tuning up your heart rate can offer an array of positive promises that, unlike the commercials on television, can deliver fulfillment, enjoyment, and a longer, happier life. In fact, I often refer to exercise and physical activity as a "magic pill."

If you could design a magic pill to do anything you wanted, what would you choose? Most doctors and patients want a pill that achieves the desired effect, has few side effects, and is convenient as well as affordable.

A survey of my patients and my seminar audiences revealed that they wanted a pill that would help them do the following:

- Lose weight
- Feel better
- Decrease their blood pressure
- Have more energy
- Improve their sex lives

Pleasurable Pursuits

- Prevent heart attacks
- Prevent cancer
- Look younger
- Prevent strokes
- Build stronger bones
- Prevent osteoporosis
- Improve mood and prevent depression

Regular physical activity is that magic pill! Exercise is effective in fulfilling all the above requests and is readily available and inexpensive. Since exercise has so many positive and beneficial health effects, you would expect it to be at the top of everyone's list as their most popular pastime, right? Statistics tell us otherwise. According to the "President's Council on Physical Fitness and Sports" report, only 15% of U.S. adults engage in vigorous physical activity three times a week for at least twenty minutes. Only 22% of adults get off the couch and exercise five times a week for thirty minutes. Another 25% report no physical activity at all! These statistics mean that 85% of you reading this book need to put it down, walk away from the television, and get busy exercising! I encourage you to break away from the crowd, find an activity you enjoy, and make an investment that will pay off incredible dividends. Enjoying a minimum of 30 minutes of physical activity day, three days a week, can begin to produce some of the desired effects. After your workout, you can pick up the book again and start reading. Here's some of the evidence for what exercise can do for you:

Researchers know that physical fitness is a good predictor of the risk of death.

Danish researchers studied 30,000 men and women ages 20 to 93 over a period of 14 years and published their findings in a year 2000 volume of a prestigious medical journal. Their results showed that regular exercisers were half as likely to die from any and all causes compared to their sedentary counterparts, and the greater the level of activity, the lower the risk of death for all age groups for both men and women.

Health Yourself

In short, the more fit an individual is, the lower the risk of dying from major killers such as cancer and heart attacks.

British researchers found that physical activity reduces the risk of death from all causes in men with heart disease, even if they wait until later in life to start exercising.

Equally encouraging, a survey of 24 studies in the medical literature reported in *MT* (September 1999) found that "Most cancer patients can benefit from exercise programs even while they are undergoing chemotherapy or radiation treatment." Dr. Kerry Cournyea, author of the study, found that physical activity contributed to improvements in physical functioning and quality of life for cancer patients as well as enhancing their physical strength and endurance (*Annals of Behavioral Medicine*, 1999).

A report from the Cooper Institute in Dallas presented at the 2000 meeting of the American College of Sports Medicine also suggested that men with higher levels of fitness are less likely to die from cancer. Cooper Clinic researchers found that men who flunked their treadmill stress tests were 80% more likely to die from cancer than their more fit counterparts.

These doctors also found that a man's fitness level is an important factor in his risk of dying from lung cancer. Even in smokers, the higher the level of fitness, the lower the risk of dying from lung cancer. Of course, the risk of dying from lung cancer can be reduced drastically by never starting to smoke or by stopping tobacco use altogether.

By the same token, you don't have to be an Olympic athlete to enjoy the benefits of increased physical activity. Moderate exertion on a regular basis can help you live longer and better. Even those who have been lifelong couch potatoes can reverse their health risks by starting to exercise. Even one 45-minute session on a treadmill can lower blood pressure significantly and the results can last up to 24 hours.

Attention employers:: Employees who participate in employer-sponsored health promotion and physical fitness activities lose fewer days of work due to disability, have lower rates of employee turnover, and nearly 25% less

Pleasurable Pursuits

health care costs than those who do not participate in such programs. As you will see throughout this section on exercise, physical activity can improve musculoskeletal strength and flexibility and these effects can lower the rate of injury and disability. In short, regular exercise leads to an improved sense of well being, improved productivity, and lower rates of absenteeism.

Physical activity is the strongest predictor of total body fat and central abdominal fat, both of which are associated with a higher risk of health problems. Experts say that being fat is due more to inactivity than to genetics. While regular exercise and activity may result in less weight loss than you had hoped for, measuring success in the battle of the bulge requires more than just reading the scales. Modest weight loss may result in more energy, a better self-image, and an increased level of fitness. You don't have to be skinny to be healthy, either. Overweight individuals who exercise have a better risk profile than normal weight individuals who are less physically active. To determine your degree of health risk based on you weight, use the following chart to measure your BMI, or Body Mass Index. Find the place on the chart where your height and weight intersect. The number in that column is your BMI reading. The optimal BMI range for men and women is 26-28. If you have a BMI over 30, you are considered obese and at risk for developing severe health consequences such as heart disease and diabetes. The higher the BMI, the higher the health risk. If you already have risk factors such as diabetes or high blood pressure, a BMI above 27 is the lower limit of the danger zone.

Do you know your own BMI?

height \ weight	120	130	140	150	160	170	180	190	200	210	220	230	240	250
5'0"	23	25	27	29	31	33	35	37	39	41	43	45	47	49
5'2"	22	23	26	27	29	31	33	35	37	38	40	42	44	46
5'4"	21	22	24	26	28	29	31	33	34	36	38	40	41	43
5'6"	19	21	23	24	26	27	29	31	32	34	36	37	39	40
5'8"	18	20	21	23	24	26	27	29	30	32	34	35	37	38
5'10"	17	19	20	22	23	24	26	27	29	30	32	33	35	36
6'0"	16	18	19	20	22	23	24	26	27	29	30	31	33	34
6'2"	15	17	18	19	21	22	23	24	26	27	28	30	31	32

Health Yourself

Never Too Young

Young people can benefit from increasing their level of activity as well, but their participation statistics aren't much better than those of adults. Only 50% of young people ages 12 to 21 are involved in vigorous physical activity. Only 25% perform light to moderate activity, and the remaining 25% don't exercise at all!

Those who exercise regularly drastically lower their odds of developing diabetes as adults. They also improve their chances of maintaining a normal weight. A physically active child usually becomes an active adult who reaps the many benefits we discuss in this section.

For example, teenage physical activity appears to reduce the risk of breast cancer in certain individuals. Women who were physically active as teenagers had a 44% risk reduction of breast cancer later in life, and three or more hours per week of physical activity as a teenager is associated with an average six- to eight-year delay in the onset of breast cancer once a woman reaches age 50.

Likewise, moderate activity such as an hour of brisk walking a day can reduce the risk of developing type-2 (non-insulin dependent) diabetes by half (*FPN*, September 1, 2001).

Another study showed that even low intensity exercise lessens the normal rise in fats in the bloodstream that occur after eating a high fat meal. Researchers in Ireland found that spending just six minutes a day climbing stairs lowers cholesterol by 15%. For every one percent reduction in cholesterol, you get a two percent reduction in the risk of a heart attack.

According to a report from the Cooper Clinic in Dallas, exercise may also help decrease the risk of duodenal (stomach) ulcers. A study of 11,000 people revealed that the most active men had a 62% reduction in ulcer risk while moderately active men had a 46% reduction (*UCBWL*).

Moderate exercise may also be enough to help prevent colon cancer, according to Harvard researchers (*Annals of Internal Medicine*, 1995).

Pleasurable Pursuits

For men, a weekly game of tennis or two to three hours of brisk walking a week "can translate into a 30% drop in the risk of developing colon cancer."

Tee It Up for Your Health

Compared to sedentary men, those who golfed two to three times a week for five months noted significant improvements in weight, waist size, exercise tolerance, and cholesterol levels.

A long-term study in Denmark of 30,000 men and women from 20 to 93 years of age showed that those who exercised regularly were half as likely to die from any and all causes compared to their sedentary counterparts. Norwegian researchers confirmed those findings in an article appearing in the British medical journal *Lancet*. They studied over 2,000 men ages 40 to 60 for 20 years and found a strong connection between increased fitness and a lower risk of death. The researchers found that even small improvements in fitness yielded significant improvements in longevity.

Healthy adults, the elderly, and even cardiac patients can benefit from resistance training, which develops overall health and fitness. Using free weights or resistance machines and performing up to 15 repetitions of 8 to 10 exercises at least twice a week can yield the desired benefits. As little as 30 minutes two to three times a week can be a wise investment in your health.

Researchers reported in the July 1999 issue of *Arthritis* that exercise therapy reduces pain and disability and improves function and mobility in patients with mild to moderate "wear and tear" arthritis (osteoarthritis) of the hip and knee.

For patients with congestive heart failure, regular exercise improves the function of the blood vessels supplying the circulation to the legs and increases exercise tolerance (*Circulation*, December 1998). Blood flow to the legs doubled with exercise of 25 minutes per day for six months.

Health Yourself

The elderly can get plenty of health benefits from participating in physical activity, as it prolongs life expectancy and helps to maintain independent living status by reducing the risk of falling. Activities such as gardening or walking can burn an additional 500 calories per week and lower the risk of dying by 25 to 30% in any given year.

Men and women reap the benefits of physical activity in different ways. Regular exercise lowers the risk of prostate enlargement, according to a study of over 50,000 men in the health professions. Walking two to three hours per week resulted in a 25% decrease in risk for prostate enlargement, a common condition in older men that causes frequent and difficult urination.

Stretch Away the Hot Flashes

For women, yoga stretching exercises can relieve the bothersome symptoms of menopause such as hot flashes and emotional instability. These exercises can also lead to better overall health for women, according to Susan M. Lark M.D., author of *The Estrogen Decision Self-Help Book*. Dr. Lark's research and experience shows that yoga exercises improve blood circulation, which in turn increases the level of oxygen delivered to the body's cells. Increased oxygen means more energy. Other body systems such as the digestive tract and nervous system especially benefit from these stretching activities.

Tai Chi

Once an oriental self-defense technique, Tai Chi (pronounced "tie-jee") is now a low impact form of exercise that improves balance and flexibility, reduces stress, and strengthens muscles. This slow controlled exercise form works as well as moderate aerobic exercise in lowering blood pressure, according to a 12-week-long study involving 60 subjects. Research showed that Tai Chi can also reduce blood pressure and ease arthritis symptoms (*RW*, November 2001).

Exercise can reduce the chance of death even in the face of genetic disorders. A study of twins showed that those who exercised for 30 minutes at

Pleasurable Pursuits

least six times a month had a 56% lower risk of death compared to the non-exercising twin. Even less regular occasional exercise resulted in a 30% reduction in the risk of death.

Walk Away from Heart Disease

Walking cuts the risk of heart attack 30 to 40% in women ages 40 to 65 who walk briskly at the speed of three miles per hour for at least three hours per week. Those women who spent 90 minutes a week exercising vigorously enough to induce a sweat, such as by jogging, doing heavy gardening, or housework, reduced their cardiovascular risk by 50%.

Even those women who had been sedentary and began their exercise later in life reaped the benefits of the activity. Again, researchers found that even as little exercise as one hour a week helped reduce heart attack risk.

Women over 65 years of age who exercised regularly were 36% less likely to have a hip fracture than their sedentary counterparts. Intense activities such as aerobics or weight training provided the most benefit, but women involved in less intense activities such as dancing or gardening for more than two hours a week also reaped the dividends of improved health.

Regular exercise also helped keep elderly women mentally sharp. An eight-year- long study of nearly 6,000 women age 65 and older found that those who exercised the most were the least likely to experience a decline in their mental function (*FPN*, November 2001).

Honey, I Got the Exercise

Experts at the University of Memphis recommend eating three tablespoons of honey immediately prior to exercise. Eating the honey plain or putting it in tea (see the section on tea for its benefits) provides a steady flow of energy during a strenuous workout, and honey affects your blood sugar less radically than other forms of carbohydrates such as sweets and sodas.

Health Yourself

Brain researchers suggest that an invigorating walk gives older peoples' brains a good workout, resulting in improved memory and sharper judgment, according to an article in a 2000 issue of the journal *Nature*. Even those who had been previously inactive benefited from the increased activity. After six months of walking for an hour three times a week, the study subjects, men and women ages 60 to 75, showed improvement in "executive control processes" such as scheduling, planning, and responding to changing circumstances.

Experts are beginning to discover how exercise causes these changes to occur. Researchers at the Salk Institute and Princeton University found that regular running and intensive mental exercise revitalize the mind by stimulating the growth of new brain cells responsible for learning and memory. Physical activity also measurably improved the survival of existing brain cells, especially in the part of the brain involved in memory function. Previous studies also showed exercise may reduce the risk of developing Alzheimer's disease later in life.

Here's good news for regular joggers: you are at no greater risk of developing arthritis and other bone ailments than people who do not exercise. Even runners in their sixties show no more wear and tear than couch potatoes the same age.

Here's more good news: exercise combined with a low-fat vegetarian diet can reverse blockage in the circulation of the heart without using any of the usual medications. Other benefits include weight loss and improved cholesterol levels.

Beating the Blues

Canadian researchers reviewed all the medical studies on exercise and mental health published since 1981 and found that all forms of exercise helped alleviate mild to moderate depression and were also effective in patients with anxiety and substance abuse problems. In one 1999 Canadian study of seriously depressed patients, those who ran, walked, or did strength

Pleasurable Pursuits

training exercises three times a week for 20 to 60 minutes at a time showed significant improvements in their symptoms of depression. These improvements lasted up to a year. Exercising 10 minutes a day for four weeks also improved the mood and mental outlook in college women, according to a study in the journal *Health Psychology* reported in *RW*.

Exactly how exercise works to relieve anxiety and depression is unknown, but researchers think it may be due to the release of brain chemicals such as endorphins, which are natural antidepressants. Exercise reduces stress, which may account for some of its beneficial effects.

A study of 135 college students showed that those who exercised handled stress better than those who were less active. By reducing the physical symptoms of stress, exercise also decreased the risk of heart attacks, ulcers, and strokes. Stress is a "magnifying glass" that can worsen conditions such as arthritis and chronic pain. Leisure time physical activity buffers these effects of stress and leads to an overall better mood and higher quality of life. Another study showed that college students who exercised regularly were better equipped to handle life's stresses and had fewer physical symptoms of stress than their less active counterparts.

Never Too Old

Weight training improved moods for elderly exercisers more than any other form of physical activity, according to researchers who analyzed 32 different studies of men and women ages 62 and up. Experts say that weight training produces the most effect because the payoff comes quickly. Older people who exercise reported better moods than those who were out of shape, and studies suggest that younger people can get the same benefits.

Weight training builds muscle that "edges out" fat, speeds up metabolism, and helps the body use insulin "more efficiently," according to an article in the July 1995 issue of *Hippocrates*. The same article also says you will see a 20% increase in muscle strength within just three months of starting a weight training program.

Health Yourself

Studies show that burning an additional 500 calories per week (the equivalent of walking five miles) can lower the risk of death in the elderly by 25 to 35%. Other benefits include lower blood pressure, lower risk of falls and fractures, and prevention of osteoporosis.

A 65-year-old woman today can expect to live another 16 years, and staying active can improve her quality of life and delay the need for assisted living or custodial care.

Dodging the Knife

Exercise may result in fewer gallbladder operations. Women who exercised 30 minutes a day five times a week cut their risk of developing gallbladder disease by 20% while physically active middle-aged men reduced their risk by 50%. Researchers think the effects of exercise upon cholesterol, body fat, and insulin provides the protection. Regular exercise could thus make an impact on the 800,000 hospitalizations per year for gallbladder surgery. At the same time, men who watched over 40 hours of television per week had double the risk of developing gallstone symptoms compared to those watching fewer than six hours of TV per week.

Exercise – A Stroke of Genius

Physical activity also reduces the risk of stroke, according to a study of 11,000 college alumni. Men who exercised at the level of 1,000 to 2,000 calories per week (walking a mile = 100 calories) had a 40% reduction in stroke risk compared to those who did little or no exercise. Burning up to 1,000 calories per week by exercising decreases stroke risk up to 46%, but there was no additional benefit beyond that level of exercise, according to an article in the medical journal *Stroke* (October 1998). Another 10-year study from Iceland, reported in a 1999 issue of the *Annals of Internal Medicine*, found that the risk of stroke was 31% lower in men who remained physically active after the age of 40 compared to their sedentary peers.

Pleasurable Pursuits

Remaining physically active after age 40 also protects men against stroke, according to a recent study. Stroke risk was reduced by 31% in men who stayed physically active after age 40 compared to their couch potato peers. The type of physical activity performed did not make any difference in the outcome, although there was a suggestion that low-intensity activities such as walking account for most of the protective effect.

It may be that exercise protects against strokes by lowering blood pressure. Research reported in *FPN* (June 1995) found that a brisk walk three to four times a week for 30 to 40 minutes can have a significant impact on lowering blood pressure.

Physical activity, including moderate exercise such as walking, substantially reduced women's risk of stroke as well. The more time they spent exercising, the lower the risk of stroke for the women who participated in the study. Those who exercised almost 22 hours per week had a 44% lower risk of stroke than those who spent less than two hours per week in physical activity.

Clearly, when it comes to exercise, more is better. Scientists showed that exercise promotes atheroprotective factors, the "good guys" that protect circulation, while reducing atherogenic factors, the "bad guys" that block circulation and cause strokes and heart attacks.

The good news is that the higher your fitness level, the higher your level of protection. Our only limit is the body's capacity to perform, which can improve with training.

Cancer Protection

Most experts agree that regular physical activity reduces the risk of colon cancer and may also lower the risk of breast cancer.

Recent research suggests that men with high fitness levels are less likely to die from cancer. Men who were unfit and obese had an almost three-fold increase in their risk of dying from cancers of the colon, prostate, kidney, and lung due to the dangers of too much body fat.

Health Yourself

The American Cancer Society encourages people to follow the U.S. Surgeon General's advice to get 30 minutes of mild to moderate activity three to five days per week.

A survey of 24 research projects reported in the medical literature revealed that many cancer patients benefit from exercise programs while receiving radiation or chemotherapy treatments.

This review of the research in the September 1999 issue of *Medical Tribune* consistently found that "exercise contributed to improvements in physical functioning and quality of life of cancer patients as well as improving their physical strength and endurance."

Exercise – The Anti-Aging Machine

Aging is a complex process that is highly variable between individuals. Even different organs and systems in the same person may age at different rates. Genetics, lifestyle, immune system, and disease processes determine a person's rate of aging. Poor health and frailty are not the natural consequences of the aging process. Although we cannot yet alter our genetic makeup, we can make healthy lifestyle choices that reduce our risk of disabling diseases later in life and help ensure that we "die young as late in life as possible." Regular exercise and physical activity are choices that can lead to healthy, successful, and productive aging.

For men, the percentage of body fat increases from an average of 15% to 35 to 40% between the ages of 20 and 80. Body fat in women doubles from 20 to 40% in the same time frame. Exercise reduces body fat, improves the overall level of fitness, and lessens the chance of falls and injuries by protecting against muscular weakness. There is no age limit for exercise and it's never too late to start. Exercisers live longer and healthier lives, have better appetites and digestion, and experience fewer sleep disturbances and less depression.

Experts tell us that the average person experiences a one percent decline in aerobic fitness each year. Doing the math tells us that between ages 30 and 60, there is a 30% decrease in overall fitness levels. Recent studies proved that a three-month program of moderate intensity exercise can potentially boost aerobic fitness levels by 15 to 20%. By engaging in such a program, a 60-year-old couch potato could regain the fitness level of a 40- to 45-year-old (*Patient Care*, November 1999).

Rusting Out

The process of producing the energy required to carry out bodily functions is known as "oxidation" and it produces dangerous compounds known as free radicals. The name sounds like some kind of extreme student activist during the 1960s, but instead, these are compounds that damage the cells in our bodies through a reaction known as oxidative stress. When rust forms on metal, that's an oxidative process, and you've seen what rust can do to even the strongest metal. The same thing goes on in every cell of our bodies every day. Certain dietary fats, tobacco use, alcohol, and environmental pollutants act to increase the negative effects of oxidative stress. Antioxidants are chemicals that act as scavengers, much like vitamins E and C, and protect the body from free radicals. Increasing the level of antioxidants, by exercising or enjoying certain foods and beverages, counteracts the effects of the free radicals and helps reverse the aging process.

Exercise – Don't Leave Home to Get It

Should you do your exercise at home or pack your bags and head to the local fitness club or YMCA? Interestingly enough, researchers have found that exercisers at home are more likely to maintain their participation and lose more weight than those who participate in group activities. However, the choice is a highly personal one and my advice is to do what works best for you. Part of the exercise experience for me is the opportunity to visit and socialize with the other gym regulars. My friend Ann is just the opposite, preferring the privacy of her own home or the quiet of solitary walks through the woods.

Health Yourself

Fit or Fat?

Don't get discouraged if your exercise program doesn't get you down to your ideal weight. Being overweight and fit is healthier than being thin and unfit. In one study, the fit participants had lower death rates from all causes compared to their unfit counterparts, regardless of weight. Take the advice of the experts in a 1999 volume of the *Journal of Clinical Nutrition*, who advise us to focus on overall health and fitness rather than on the weight reading of the scales.

Your Own Exercise Prescription

You can write your own exercise prescription when you understand the basics contained in the abbreviation "FIT."

F = Frequency, or how often you exercise. Most experts agree that performing physical activity at least three and optimally five days per week is necessary to achieve most of the health benefits of exercise. Rest days are important in preventing injury and avoiding burnout. Going too far too fast can result in injury or burnout and take you from being a couch potato to being an "ouch" potato and short circuit your good intentions.

I = Intensity, or how hard you work out. Fitness experts measure the degree of exercise by monitoring heart rates. Subtracting your age from 220 is a rough estimate of your maximum heart rate. Ideally, your exercise should keep you at 75 to 85% of your maximum heart rate. Counting your pulse for 10 seconds and multiplying by six will give you your heart rate per minute. Another "quick and dirty" method of assessing exercise intensity is known as the "talk test." If you are too short-winded to carry on a normal conversation while you are exercising, your level of exertion is probably too high. You can also buy electronic heart rate monitors from fitness stores and catalogs.

T = Time, refers to the duration of your workout session. The ideal workout session is thirty minutes long, but beginners may need to start with shorter sessions and gradually increase their exercise time. If you are

Pleasurable Pursuits

unable to do 30 minutes at once, it is equally effective to divide your time into 10- or 15-minute segments two or three times a day.

Building up to one full hour of exercise will provide an extra payoff for those trying to lose weight. Researchers found that exercising for an hour keeps the body's metabolism rate revved up for the next eight hours, so you burn up calories long after the hour of exercise is done!

Workout Guidelines

Beginners should always consult a physician before starting an exercise program. I usually recommend doing 10 minutes of light to moderate exercise three times a week.

Warming up with stretching or calisthenics for five minutes before starting your activity can reduce the chance of injury. Then exercise with enough intensity to maintain your heart rate at the target level for 10 minutes followed by five minutes of cool down and stretching.

Each week, add another minute of exercise to your routine.

For even greater benefits, build up to 45 minutes four to five times a week and choose exercises from the following list of activities in the chart below.

Activities

Light to moderate activities (these burn calories and oxygen at three to six times the level of the inactive body):

Brisk walking (three to four miles per hour)

Swimming

Bicycle riding (six to 10 miles per hour)

Table tennis

Golfing (pulling your clubs)

Health Yourself

Fly fishing (casting while standing)

Canoeing (two to four miles per hour)

Lawn mowing or yard work

Housework, general cleaning

Vigorous Activities:

Power walking (four to five miles per hour)

Cycling (over 10 miles per hour)

Swimming (faster)

Stair climbing or cross-country ski machines

Canoeing (over five miles per hour)

Yard work with a push mower

Heavy moving (furniture)

These calculations were based on women with an average weight of 129 pounds. In general, the more one weighs, the more calories one will burn during exercise.

EXERCISE MACHINE	CALORIES BURNED IN 20 MINUTES		
Intensity	Low	Moderate	High
Treadmill	190	222	234
Rower	166	198	230
Cross-country skier	178	194	212
Stair stepper	114	174	196
Stationary bike	92	132	172
Rider	114	132	146

Pleasurable Pursuits

Exorcising Your Excuses

> *"If God had intended us to exercise, he would have given us better knees."*
>
> Anonymous

"Yes, but…" are two of the deadliest words in the English language. Patients say "Yes, but" all the time when I suggest exercise. Over the years I have heard just about every excuse for why a person can't exercise. When I bring up the idea of exercise, my patients seem to be very creative in coming up with excuses for not participating and following my recommendations.

I say something like, "Mrs. Higgins, if you would go for a walk regularly you might be able to stop some of your blood pressure medications."

Patients like Mrs. Higgins often reply, *"Yes, but my knees won't let me"* or *"Yes, but I'm too tired."*

I remind the complainers that there are non-weight-bearing exercises such as water aerobics that spare aching joints like hips and knees from the pounding of activities such as running and walking. Most people need help understanding that their lack of exercise is the reason for their fatigue. I also remind them that when they begin to enjoy the activities of their choice, one of the end results will be that they actually have *more* energy.

"I get plenty of exercise at work" is another common refrain. When I ask my patients about exercise, many of them respond that since they are physically active at work, they don't feel the need to participate in exercise during their off-work leisure hours.

This notion is wrong, according to Italian researchers who studied thousands of workers over 10 years. Their studies showed that physical activity performed during leisure time resulted in multiple health benefits but on-the-job "exercise" did not.

Specifically, the physical activity performed away from work was related to an improvement in insulin resistance in adults. Insulin is the hormone that

Health Yourself

controls the blood sugar level and is involved in other chemical reactions in the body. Insulin resistance occurs when cells lose their sensitivity to the hormone leading to weight gain and elevated cholesterol, both of which are risk factors for diabetes and heart disease. Exercise reduces insulin resistance and protects against two of the major causes of premature death: heart attacks and diabetes.

Researchers think the reason on-the-job exercise is not as beneficial is that it is not as intensive as after hours-physical activity. They suggest that perhaps, "People exert themselves more at play."

I will list some of the other common excuses I hear and take the air out of *your* favorite reason for not exercising:

"Doc, it's dark when I leave for work and dark when I get home…I just don't have time to work out or exercise." To these people I say, "You have plenty of time; you just choose to spend it in other activities." Exercise takes time, but not as much as you think. Committing 30 minutes three times a week is a good start. That's less than two hours a week, and most of us spend more time than that watching television. It's simply a matter of setting your priorities and investing time in yourself and your health. People who don't have time to exercise always seem to have time for illness and disability!

"Doc, it's way too late for me to start exercising. I'm too old." Many of us think that declining mobility, strength, and endurance are effects of aging, but these effects are actually due to our inactivity and are *reversible*. One group of nursing home patients whose average age was 87 (nearly a third were 90 years old) participated in a research study using exercise machines for 45 minutes three times a week for 12 weeks to strengthen their legs. When they completed the study, the exercisers increased their walking speed by 12% and improved their stair-climbing ability by 28%. Four of the group members were dependent upon walkers to get around, but after the exercise program they were able to walk using only a cane. Two exercisers who used canes were able to walk without using any assistance at all! Those who exercised experienced less depression and were more likely to be independent and participate in nursing-home activities. It's never too late to start!

Pleasurable Pursuits

"Doc, I'd rather have a root canal than exercise." Many of us have the ABE syndrome (Anything But Exercise) and would rather spend our time in less active pursuits. We prefer working on the computer, listening to music, reading, conversing, or anything except exercise! For those who invoke this excuse I have a suggestion: find an activity you enjoy and combine it with one of your non-exercise activities. Listen to tapes or read while you walk on the treadmill or ride the stationary bike. Safety experts remind us to not use headphones while jogging or riding outside.

"Doc, I'm not putting on a swimsuit or wearing those shorts." I hear this mostly from women who say they are embarrassed to wear their exercise attire in public. I am living proof that you don't have to look like an athlete to suit up and exercise. I work out at the gym every day and when I see a woman or a man with a less than athletic physique I think more about how great it is that they are there working out than about their appearance. There are enough of us around that we constitute the majority and we don't worry what we look like.

"Doc, I'm too tired." This is the most common excuse I hear and it's the easiest to dispel. My personal experience confirms the claim that expending energy creates more energy. I tell people that the reason they don't have energy is that they don't exercise. Once you get into a routine of exercise, you will find your overall level of energy will increase.

Exercise – The Bottom Line

"Exercise might be a pretty powerful instrument for sexual enhancement" say researchers at the University of San Diego. These scientists put 78 middle-aged men on an aerobic exercise program for an hour three times a week for nine months. Exercising at 75 to 80% of their maximum ability, these men reported having more and more satisfying sex and orgasms than before. They also reported that their bodies functioned better sexually than before.

The bottom line is, physical activity can pump up your sex life! Exercise leads to improved endurance and other changes in the body such as increased testosterone levels that improve sexuality; it may also improve heart function.

Caution: Overdoing exercise can have a negative effect on your love life if you spend so much time on exercising that you ignore your partner. Also, excessive workouts can lower sex hormone levels, causing a reduced sex drive in men and menstrual difficulties for women.

The Sex Prescription – Let's Get It On

PRO-vention is all about enjoyable activities that can improve your health, and sex certainly qualifies as a pleasurable pursuit. Most of you are probably more familiar with the pleasurable aspects of a satisfying sex life than with its physical and emotional benefits. "Let's get it on" and explore some of the science behind the health benefits of sexual pleasure.

Oddly enough, it was British researchers who first studied the effects of sex on health! They found that among women, those who had more frequent and satisfying sexual encounters were less likely to have heart trouble. Men who reported more frequent and more satisfying sex lives had an overall lower death rate than those who had less frequent and less satisfying sex. U.S. research experts didn't want the British to have all the fun, so Americans began to look into the subject as well. Sexuality expert and author Laura Corn outlines many of these research articles in her excellent book and audiotape, *The Great American Sex Diet.* One of Ms. Corn's references is Dr. Michael Rozien's book *Real Age*, in which he notes that the average frequency of sexual activity in the United States is once a week. Married people have more sex than singles, and frequency also varies with age, economic status, educational level, and ethnic background. Dr. Rozien found that if you have sex twice a week, you lower your risk age by almost two years. That means your health risks are the same as for someone two years younger than you. If you increase your frequency of sex to five to seven times a week and are happy with your sex life, you decrease your risk age by almost eight years. Sex really can make you younger! So why be average? We have a patriotic duty to uphold American superiority in the sexual Olympics!

Pleasurable Pursuits

According to a survey published in the December 2001 *Chicago Tribune*, Americans have sex 124 times a year to lead all other nations. Greeks occupy second place in the sexual frequency derby at 117 times a year, while South Africans and New Zealanders are in a dead heat for third place with a lovemaking frequency of 116 and 115 times a year respectively.

In Ms. Corn's tape one of my favorites quotes is from Graham Masterton's *How to Make Love Six Nights a Week*: "Having frequent sex does very much more than release tension. It raises your self-esteem, re-establishes closeness with your partner, defines your status as a woman, and demonstrates that somebody needs you and desires you. Frequent sex is good for your self-confidence. Frequent sex improves your physical fitness and general well-being. Frequent sex gives you a positive, more creative attitude toward life and has a direct beneficial effect on anything you are trying to accomplish at home or at work. Frequent sex makes you calm and less irritable, improves your self-image, and allows you to explore the full potential of your body, your emotions, and your imagination. Without a doubt, frequent sex can change your life from top to bottom."

If you are one of the 24 million American women who have low sexual desire (as reported in *JAMA* (1999)), you may benefit from following Ms. Corn's advice in *The Great American Sex Diet*. Low sexual desire occurs in 22% of women and five percent of men; in women sexual problems decrease with age while in men, increasing age means an increase in sexual difficulties. Both men and women who increase their frequency of satisfying sex may experience some of the other benefits such as a stronger immune system to fight off infections. Other benefits of more frequent and satisfying sex include improved sleep, better digestion, and fewer menstrual cramps for women. After menopause, women may be able to avoid some of the accompanying physical problems such as hot flashes.

Bedroom activity may also improve your learning ability and memory. Because of the intensity of sexual stimulation, it triggers chemical changes in the brain that result in more connections between brain cells. Neurological experts tell us that the more connections we have, the more capacity we have to learn and remember new things.

Health Yourself

Also, when we make love more often our bodies reduce the output of cortisol, the stress hormone that can lead to fatigue and increased cravings and binges.

An unusual health benefit occurred in Israel when a man with hiccups tried every known cure and folk remedy without results. His hiccups suddenly disappeared after he had sexual intercourse and an intense orgasm.

Besides all the other benefits, having more and better sex leads to…well, more and better sex, which in turn leads to…well, you get the picture!

An article in *Redbook* magazine (May 2000) says, "If you want hotter sex, bypass the bedroom and head straight for the kitchen." Here's the scoop on eight foods that may improve your love life!

1. Honey. The sweet sticky stuff is a bountiful source of boron, a trace mineral that is involved in the metabolism of estrogen, the primary female sex hormone. Dr. Theresa Crenshaw, author of *The Alchemy of Love and Lust,* says that boron may also boost levels of testosterone, the hormone that stimulates the drive for sex and orgasms in men and women.

2. Walnut oil. You may learn to look at cholesterol differently when you realize it's the basis for all sex hormones! Following a rigorous non-fat diet can lower your levels of sex hormones and thus trigger a reduction in your sex drive. Fats from vegetables, nuts, and seeds can provide the fatty acids your body needs to manufacture sex hormones and jump-start your libido. "Cold-pressed" oils such as walnut oil are higher in nutrients and vitamin E than heat-processed oils.

3. Oats. Eating a cup of oatmeal three times a week increases the level of the sex hormone testosterone in the bloodstream.

4. Oysters. The classic aphrodisiac featured in the movie *Tom Jones* may deserve its reputation due to the high level of minerals that are key ingredients in sex hormones.

5. Kelp. Loss of libido in some women may be due to an undetectable low level of thyroid hormone. Seaweed is rich in iodine and sprinkling dried

Pleasurable Pursuits

kelp over salads or rice may yield noticeable results after a month of regular use. Once the thyroid kicks in, the libido soon follows.

6. Chocolate. This sensuous treat derives some of its pleasurable sensations from the methylxanthines, chemicals essential to the nervous system that also create a feeling of satisfaction. Chocolate belongs to a class of foods called "organoleptics" whose properties of texture, color, and scent help get us in the mood for love.

7. Eggs. Pantothenic acid and vitamin B-6 are found in abundance in eggs and help maintain your body's hormone balance, keep your energy level up, and improve your ability to handle stress.

8. Steak. Lean red meats contain zinc, a trace metal that lowers the production of the pituitary hormone prolactin that at higher levels can cause sexual problems. Other sources of zinc include dark meat poultry, seafood, whole grains, brown rice, and green leafy vegetables. Zinc may keep the zing in your sex life!

Additional Pleasurable Pursuits

There are other pleasurable pursuits that can help keep you healthy, too. Why not try a few and see what happens?

Imagine That!

Medical experts are beginning to recognize the benefits of using mental imagery and visualization to produce calming, energizing, or healing responses in your body. Specifically, sports researchers have shown that using sexual imagery is very effective against pain. In one study, college students were subjected to pain and half the group were instructed to use sexual fantasy to take their mind off the pain. The sexual fantasy group tolerated the pain twice as long as the non-fantasizers, handled the pain better, and had less anxiety, depression, and anger.

Health Yourself

Put It in Writing

Writing about your life may improve your health and help you lose weight. Researchers found that 50% of patients with chronic asthma or arthritis experienced a reduction in their symptoms after writing about their traumatic events in a journal.

Weight-loss experts found that keeping a food diary or journal increases your chances of reaching your weight-loss goals. Such writing is not intended to be a work of literary achievement. Content, spelling, and grammar take a back seat to just jotting down your thoughts and feelings on a regular basis.

Meditate on It

Adding "guided meditation" to the usual treatment of psoriasis resulted in faster clearing of the skin. Meditation and relaxation techniques also have beneficial effects for patients with chronic pain or heart disease. Regular meditation lowers stress levels and blood pressure that in turn may reduce the chances of developing hardening of the arteries.

A six- to nine-month program of transcendental meditation led to a decrease in hardening of the arteries in African-American patients with high blood pressure, leading to a decreased risk of heart attack and stroke.

Researchers at UCLA's medical school taught stress reduction techniques like deep breathing and listening to relaxation tapes to a group of high blood pressure patients and 73% were able to reduce their medication, while more than half were able to stop their medication altogether.

Please Rub It In

Regular therapeutic massage not only makes you feel relaxed, it may also improve your body's immune system. One study suggests that parents can improve their child's asthma, insomnia, diabetes, or skin disorders by giving

Pleasurable Pursuits

daily 15- to 20-minute massages, which reduce stress and improve the function of the body's immune (defense) system. In children with asthma, massage therapy decreased anxiety and improved lung function. Young insomniacs were more than twice as likely to improve with massage therapy.

Giving yourself hand and ear massages can reduce or possibly eliminate nicotine cravings, according to an article from *Preventive Medicine*. Circular motion and pressure reduced cigarette consumption from 16 per day to one a day.

Massage therapy even showed benefits for premature infants: 15 minutes of massage three times a day for 10 days led to 47% more weight gain and six fewer days in the hospital at a savings of $10,000 per infant. For full-term infants, 15 minutes of massage over six weeks (compared to rocking) resulted in increased activity and alertness, lower stress hormones, falling asleep easier, greater weight gain, and increased social interaction.

For pregnant women, 30 minutes of massage twice a week for four weeks (compared to relaxation therapy) yielded lower levels of anxiety and depression, lower stress hormones, less sleep disturbance, lower childbirth complications, and lower rates of premature births.

Massage during the childbirth process (compared to standard breathing exercises) resulted in lower anxiety and depression, lower stress hormones, less medication, shorter labor, a decreased hospital stay, and less post-partum depression.

For patients suffering from lower back pain, 30 minutes of massage twice a week for five weeks decreased pain symptoms compared to those who used muscle relaxation and also resulted in improved range of motion, less anxiety and depression, and an overall improved mood.

Migraine headache sufferers who had 30 minutes of massage twice a week for four weeks compared to standard medical treatment noticed fewer distressing symptoms, less pain, more headache-free days, better sleep, and less medication usage.

Health Yourself

For diabetic children, 15 minutes of massage a day for 30 days yielded improved insulin and food regulation and lower blood sugar levels compared to standard medical therapy alone.

For asthmatic children, 20 minutes of massage at bedtime by parents for 30 days compared to standard care led to decreased anxiety, improved mood, fewer asthma attacks, and improved lung function.

HIV positive adults who received massage for 45 minutes daily for a month showed improvement in certain immune functions compared to those receiving standard treatments.

Stage I and II breast cancer patients who underwent massage for 45 minutes three times a week for five weeks experienced improved immune function, less anxiety, pain, and anger, and improved mood and body awareness.

Teenage psychiatric patients who received massage for 30 minutes twice a week for four weeks had less depression and anxiety, lower stress hormones, and better sleep compared to those using relaxation tapes.

Patients with eating disorders such as bulimia and anorexia who received 30 minutes of massage twice a week for four weeks had less depression and anxiety and improved eating habits and body image, compared to those who received only standard medical therapy.

ZZZZZzzzz

Sleep is certainly a pleasurable activity for many of us, and warming up your toes can help you get to sleep easier and faster. The width of the blood vessels in your hands and feet determines how much time you require to fall asleep. Specifically, heat causes your blood vessels to dilate or expand and thus reduces the time required to nod off.

Sleep is important, but how much is enough? According to experts, people who get only seven hours of sleep per night live longer than those

Pleasurable Pursuits

who sleep eight hours or more per night (*FPN*, 1998). Regular use of sleeping pills was associated with a higher risk of death in one study.

By the way, researchers recently looked at whether regular exercise could prevent or treat sleep disorders such as difficulty falling or staying asleep, daytime drowsiness, and nightmares. In a study of over 700 men and women, those who exercised regularly had a reduced risk of sleep disorders.

Animal House

High blood pressure patients with pets had lower pressures and stress levels than those treated with medication alone. Heart attack patients with pets had a lower chance of having a repeat attack than those without pets.

Research also shows that couples who own cats or dogs have healthier relationships than couples who don't have a pet. Blood pressure and heart rate levels were measured under stress conditions between spouses; couples with pets had lower readings and a quicker return to normal levels than those without pets.

Austrian scientists found that frequent contact with farm animals during childhood may provide lifetime protection against allergies. Children living on farms and frequently exposed to animals were only one-third as sensitive to developing allergic symptoms compared to those living in non-rural settings.

Researchers at the Medical College of Georgia, Augusta, followed 473 children and found that those who were exposed to two or more pets in the first year of life had fewer allergies to pets, dust mites, ragweed, and grass when skin tested at slightly less than seven years of age.

Chew on This

I know, I know; we're not supposed to chew gum in public, but at least some of us might want to consider chewing gum a little more often regardless of where we are. Why? Chewing gum may relieve the symptoms of stomach irritation caused by excessive acid production. In another study, researchers found that chewing gum burned up enough calories to cause weight loss of up to 11 pounds a year.

Caution: Aspartame, the artificial sweetener in sugarless gum, may induce migraine headaches in susceptible patients. Sorbitol, the other sweetener, may cause diarrhea.

Something's Fishy Here

Placing tanks of brightly colored fish in nursing homes had positive effects such as increased relaxation and alertness for Alzheimer's patients. The aquariums held the patients' attention for up to 30 minutes – a relatively long attention span for Alzheimer's patients. This study also showed a decrease in episodes of disruptive behavior and a 20% increase in food intake for those who viewed the fish tanks.

Researchers suggest that these effects can lead to lower overall health care costs by reducing the need for nutritional supplements and medications to control behavior. No research has been done on the effects of having aquariums at home, but it would not be surprising to expect similar results.

You Deserve a Break Today

Do you crave a nap on a lazy Sunday afternoon but feel it would be too indulgent? Think again. Men who take regular naps are 50% less likely to have a heart attack than those men who do not nap regularly. Half-hour naps reduce risks by 30% and one-hour naps reduce risks by 50%. Unfortunately, naps longer than one hour produce no benefit.

A Night on the Town

Attending cultural events such as live theatre, concerts, movies, and sporting events can increase longevity. Those who attend 80 such events a year

Pleasurable Pursuits

live longer than those who attend only half as many events per year. Reading and singing activities decrease the risk of death, but not to the extent that cultural activities do. Activities such as attending religious services and going to the movies, restaurants, and sporting events are as important as physical exercise for increasing survival in the elderly, according to another study in *The British Medical Journal*.

Get Out of Town

Taking regular vacations is associated with a longer, healthier life according to recent research. Vacations, sleep, exercise, and other leisure activities appear to be restorative and protective against the negative effects of psychological stress. Researchers found that over a nine-year span, men who took vacations in most of those years were 20% less likely to die from any cause than those men who took no time off. Vacationers were also 30% less likely to die from heart disease. So, taking a couple of weeks off from work every year can make a big difference in your health.

Catch a Friend, Not a Cold

Being around lots of different people may protect you from the ravages of the common cold. Research published in the *MBHN* (1998) tells us that the more diverse your set of social contacts, the less likely you are to catch a cold. Expanding your network of friends, family, co-workers, neighbors, and fellow members of religious and community organizations to six contacts every two weeks results in less risk of illness than those who have only one to three relationships in the same time period. The total number of people is not as important as the diversity of contacts.

You Are My Sunshine

Researchers have found that women living in sunny climates or reporting the most sun exposure have a significantly lower risk of breast cancer. As

Health Yourself

reported by the Department of Defense Breast Cancer Research Program, exposure to sunlight for about 10 to 15 minutes per day allows the body to produce vitamin D, the chemical credited for the risk reduction. If you choose to bask in the sunlight, see the next section for practical tips on eye safety.

Look Cool So You Can Keep Looking

When you wear a baseball cap and sunglasses, you not only look cool and trendy, you protect your vision against the eye damage of cataracts. Accumulated sun exposure can result in cataracts, according to Dr. Sheila West, professor of ophthalmology at Johns Hopkins Medical School. She recommends a wide brim hat (baseball caps block about one-third of the harmful rays that cause eye damage) and sunglasses, as plastic lenses block slightly more rays than glass lenses.

While looking stylish in your hat and shades, you can grab an apple and further increase your protection against cataracts and eye damage. Apples contain a chemical called quercetin that kept the lenses of experimental animals clear even when exposed to chemicals that cause cataract formation. Quercetin belongs to a class of chemicals known as flavinoids found also in onions, broccoli, red wine, purple grape juice, and tea. An apple a day can also protect against heart disease and kidney cancer.

Sweep Stress under the Rug

Doing housework may relieve stress, according to psychology professor Dr. Michael Crabtree, who says that completing housework tasks gives you "a sense of accomplishment" that counteracts the stress that comes from incomplete tasks. Dr. Crabtree also found that gardening, yard work, and washing the car could offer the same benefits.

Pleasurable Pursuits

Chill Out with Designer Music

Music designed to have specific positive effects on listeners (designer music) may be useful in treating tension, mental distraction, and negative moods. Recent research shows that listening to designer music results in significant increases in caring, relaxation, and mental clarity. Listening to grunge rock music caused listeners to experience higher levels of hostility, sadness, tension, and fatigue, but designer music reversed these negative mood states. And, it costs little more than a song because it is a song! Researchers have also shown music assists in treating stress disorders and improves overall mental function.

Get a Whiff of This!

Stopping to smell the flowers can give you more than just a pleasant aroma. Many doctors and health professionals are using the oils extracted from plants for a variety of health benefits. In this process known as aromatherapy, the oils are inhaled, used in a bath, or placed directly on the skin. Experts are unsure as to the exact way the oils and aromas work, but they somehow stimulate the pathways between the nose and the emotional center in the brain, resulting in numerous responses including muscle relaxation.

According to Jane Buckle R.N., author of *Clinical Aromatherapy in Nursing,* aromatherapy even helps defend against fungal, bacterial, and viral infections and may one day be used as a booster for antibiotics.

In England, researchers studied more than 8,000 women in active childbirth labor and found that aromatherapy reduced the need for anesthesia. Inhaling oil of rose decreased anxiety, frankincense eased pain, and peppermint relieved nausea.

Another English study showed that elderly psychiatric patients who inhaled lavender slept as long as those who took heavy-duty sedatives – without the risk of dangerous side effects and hangover.

Health Yourself

A group of patients with a severe form of hair loss rubbed a mixture of thyme, lavender, cedarwood, and rosemary oils into their scalps once a day and 44% noted symptom improvement, compared to the 15% in the group that did not use the oils.

Cancer researchers are likewise encouraged by preliminary results showing that nausea caused by chemotherapy responds to inhaling the oils of peppermint, ginger, lavender, or mandarin.

Lower levels of postoperative stress were reported in those patients who were exposed to lavender, vanilla, and neroli fragrances at Columbia Presbyterian Hospital in New York City.

A whiff of spiced apple modifies the body's stress response by lowering blood pressure, slowing the respiratory rate, relaxing muscle tone, and slowing down the heart rate, says Dr. David Sobel in his book *Healthy Pleasures*.

Other studies have shown that inhaling pleasant aromas induces people to behave more helpfully and charitably toward others.

Conclusion

What will you choose as your pleasurable pursuits to take the place of mind-numbing pastimes such as watching television? Whether it's getting more exercise, improving or increasing your sex life, keeping a journal, using imagery or meditation, indulging in massage, getting a pet, or any of the other techniques mentioned in this section, you now have the information you need to write your own prescription for activities that are both pleasurable and healthy.

Section Three

> *All passions exaggerate: it is only because they exaggerate that they are passions.*
>
> Sebastian Chamfort

Vince Lombardi, the famous football coach, once said, "Life is an emotional game." Relationships, humor, spirituality, optimism, and altruism comprise the emotional and attitudinal aspects of life in this final section of the book, which explores how emotions, attitudes, and feelings influence our health and wellness. Sir Roger L'Estrange once said, "It is with our passions as it is with fire and water; they are good servants but bad masters." Thus, learning how to take charge of your emotions and attitudes so that they serve you rather than control you is the goal.

While this section focuses on positive passions, we cannot forget that the tapestry of the human fabric is interwoven with the fibers of negative emotions and experiences without which we could not have a fully human experience. The information presented here will not merely allow you to escape those negative passions, it will allow you to choose and have some control over your emotional life and to tip the balance toward the positive side. As Daniel Goleman tells us in his book *Emotional Intelligence*, "In the calculus of the heart it

POSITIVE PASSIONS

Health Yourself

is the ratio of positive to negative emotions that determines the sense of well-being." He continues to note the importance of attitude and emotion by saying that "Good moods, while they last, enhance the ability to think flexibly and with more complexity, making it easier to find solutions to problems, whether intellectual or interpersonal."

In this section, you will find information and data that you can use to make choices to assist you in controlling and managing your emotional life to achieve the maximum health benefit. I hope you can find something useful as you write your own prescription to health yourself. Goleman goes on to tell us, "Managing our emotions…is a full time job: much of what we do – especially in our free time – is an attempt to manage mood. Everything we choose can be a way to make ourselves feel better."

The payoff for succeeding in the arena of managing our emotions can yield positive benefits, according to author and medical expert Dr. Dean Ornish, who tells us in *Healing and the Mind* that "Most health practitioners try to motivate people to change out of fear," which Dr. Ornish says "doesn't work very well."

The purpose of the information in this section is to motivate you to change not through fear but by helping you add positive passions to your life that can "improve the joy of living" and "improve the quality and joy within your life right now."

Dr. Ornish concludes, "If you believe you have some control over your life and that you have the ability to make choices…you are more likely to make changes that are going to do you good in terms of both your behavior and the direct effect of your mind on your body."

Relationships

"Listening and being heard are important psychological nutrients that we need every day," say Anne and Charles Simpkinson in their article "Feeding One Another" (*Common Boundary*, November-December 1998). They go on to tell us, "As a nation we have the technological expertise to create

Positive Passions

highly sophisticated communications networks, but as individuals our exchanges are often primitive–even unhealthy."

According to the Simpkinsons, "The real epidemic in our culture: emotional and spiritual diseases of the heart caused by a profound sense of loneliness, isolation, alienation, and depression." Scientific evidence shows that our contacts with others are vital links in maintaining our health. A 20-year study found that "People who are isolated are at increased risk of mortality [death] from a number of causes...Social support is particularly related to survival after a myocardial infarction [heart attack]."

Research shows that our social connections not only keep us alive after heart attacks, they also defend against depression and keep our mental functions intact. These relationships may even lower the risk of getting or dying from cancer. Studies supporting these claims appeared in the *Mind/Body Health Newsletter* in 1998, which also showed that social isolation tends to have the opposite effect, making recovery from illness more difficult and resulting in increased stress hormone levels. According to the newsletter, single men 45 to 54 years of age died at twice the rate of married men the same age. Socially isolated heart attack survivors were twice as likely to die as their less isolated peers, and Harvard researcher Lisa Berkman concluded that isolation even increased the rate at which people were aging. These and other research findings support Dr. Ornish's claim that "Love, intimacy, and relationships are the most significant factors in healing."

The positive effect of social support, including close connections with caring relatives and friends, can also speed recovery from strokes and hip fractures as well as from heart attacks. Experts think that emotional support calms the patient and reduces the level of stress hormones known to bring about harmful chemical reactions in the body.

Relaxation and stress reduction reduce the risk of infection by boosting the immune system and speed up the recovery process by enhancing the chemical reactions that support healing.

Health Yourself

A Little Togetherness

Spending time together with your significant other may also have positive effects on your heart. Researchers reporting in *Psychosomatic Medicine* studied 120 healthy adults for six days and found their blood pressures were lower when they were with their sweethearts than when they were with a stranger or by themselves. A "good" marriage can have positive health benefits and a "troubled" marriage can be physically harmful. Many research studies support the previously mentioned claim that "Married people live longer than those who are single, widowed, or divorced." Widowhood and separation/divorce are linked to increased psychological problems and chronic disease, including heart disease.

Specifically, women less than 45 years of age who are divorced, separated, or widowed have higher levels of total cholesterol and LDL ("bad" cholesterol) than their married counterparts.

Men and women who find themselves in an unstable marriage headed toward separation or divorce would thus be well advised to be aware of the increased risk in this situation and to take extra measures to improve their physical and mental health.

Take Two Proverbs and Call Me in the Morning

Even mainstream medical doctors are now jumping aboard the spirituality bandwagon. Doctors who went to medical school during my era of training had little or no formal education in the realm of spirituality and religion, but "The times, they are a changin'": over 60 American medical schools now include spirituality programs in their curriculum. According to an article in the *New York Times*, "Both the religious and the medical establishments are aware of polls showing that most Americans think that faith and prayer benefit health and that doctors should discuss the connection."

Positive Passions

A nationwide survey of 438 doctors revealed that 80% of family doctors have recommended that patients seek religious counsel for help coping with grief, marital conflict, or terminal illness or dealing with substance abuse.

You may want to prescribe a healthy dose of spirituality for yourself. As the baby boomer generation ages and becomes more susceptible to health problems, the *Times* article says they are "almost as likely to elicit a spiritual quest as a search for the best specialist." Let's look at some of the research that shows why prescribing religion and spirituality as part of your lifestyle may yield positive health benefits.

According to a recent six-year study at Duke University, persons over 64 years of age who attended worship services weekly were 46% less likely to die during the six-year study compared to those whose attendance was inconsistent. The regular attendees were less likely to have depression and were quicker to seek medical care for other illnesses.

Another research project also found that regular worshippers live longer: frequent attendees lived to an average of 83 years while those who never attended services died at an average age of 73.

The Center for the Study of Religion, Spirituality, and Health at Duke University conducted studies that show deeply religious people are less likely to develop high blood pressure or depression and have stronger immune systems.

A poll of 1,000 adult Americans found that 56% said their faith had helped them recover from illness, injury, or disease.

Researchers reviewed two decades' worth of articles related to religion and health and found that in 84% of the studies, religion was associated with "clinical benefits." Another review of the medical literature found that "religious commitment may be beneficial in coping, prevention, and promoting recovery from illness."

Patients who lack social participation or religious strength and comfort are at a higher risk for complications and death following cardiac surgery.

Health Yourself

Based on the research, group participation and involvement in religious activity may improve their chances for a better recovery.

Other research bears this out: a study of over 90,000 people in Maryland indicated that death rates from heart and lung diseases were twice as high for infrequent church attendees as for those who attended church at least once a week. Likewise, a review of 18 studies on preventing heart disease found that 17 of them showed a link between religious commitment and lower rates of high blood pressure.

A study of hospitalized male patients revealed that 20% of them considered religion "the most important thing that keeps me going." Nearly 50% rated religion as "very helpful" in dealing with their illness; religious contact and activity reduced the incidence of depression in these patients.

A seven-year study of senior citizens showed religious involvement was associated with less physical disability and less depression. Plus, church attendees have nearly 50% less risk of heart attacks and have lower blood pressure than non-church goers.

Researchers also found that death rates from heart disease and emphysema were twice as high among irregular church attendees compared to those who attend once a week.

Jeffrey Levin, a researcher specializing in older adults, agrees. According to Levin, "Religious and spiritual measures…are the strongest predictors of the overall psychological well-being of older adults."

At the same time, University of Texas sociologist Robert Hummer reminds us, "The general idea isn't that religion works instant cures or that anyone who walks into a church will live to be 85, but religion is linked with many factors that benefit health over a lifetime."

Prayer Power

Lily Tomlin once remarked, "When you talk to God, it's called prayer; when God talks to you it's called schizophrenia." Many people today

Positive Passions

would take issue with that humorous assertion as they point out that communication even with higher powers is a two-way street. Regardless of whether you call it prayer, meditation, or spiritual dialogue, practicing such an activity can be beneficial to others as well as yourself.

The 1988 landmark study by Dr. Randolph Byrd opened the door on researching prayer by showing that prayer had a positive effect on patients in a coronary care unit.

Another medical journal article supported the relationship of a higher frequency of prayer activity with a higher level of mental health for those with a higher degree of physical problems.

California researchers headed by Dr. Elizabeth Targ found that prayer had some extremely beneficial effects for a group of AIDS patients: they had fewer doctor visits, fewer days in the hospital, and showed marked improvement in mood.

Prayer expert Dr. Larry Dossey recounts a story in which Bill Moyers, President Lyndon Johnson's press secretary and a former minister, was saying grace at an official lunch function. President Johnson yelled out, "Speak up, Bill; I can't hear a damn thing!"

"I wasn't addressing *you*, Mr. President," Moyers replied quietly.

Dr. Dossey sums up the growing body of research on prayer in his article "The Return of Prayer": "An impressive body of evidence suggests that prayer and religious devotion are associated with positive health outcomes

Russell Wild offers a meaningful perspective in his article in a recent issue of *Modern Maturity* magazine: "To really rev your motor, simple lifestyle changes, like regular exercise, proper nutrition, good sleep, and a positive attitude can make an immediate and intangible difference. So can taking time for spiritual and emotional fulfillment."

Dr. Wayne Muller, author of *Sabbath: Restoring the Sacred Rhythm of Rest*, says, "We need to give ourselves permission to step back and enjoy the fruits of our labors.

Health Yourself

We need to recognize that no matter how important our contributions, life continues if we stop for a while."

Muller suggests that we set aside one day a week to be "blissfully useless" while Russell Wild tells us, "You may worship if you are so inclined, or socialize with friends. But don't make business calls or balance your checkbook. Relax, and give yourself a chance to refuel."

De-Stress and Save Your Life

If you are a "hot-reactor," someone with a short fuse who flies off the handle easily, you may be setting yourself up for a stroke. Such "hot-reactors," especially men who express their anger outwardly when provoked, have an 85% higher risk of stroke over the eight years of follow-up compared to their less angry counterparts.

Researchers believe that high levels of anger and hostility are associated with the degree and progression of hardening of the arteries, which causes blockage of the blood supply to the brain, causing a stroke.

Women who bottle up their anger are more likely than other women to have a heart attack by age 60. This study showed that women who conceal their anger or are excessively concerned about their public appearance have faster heart rates, higher levels of stress hormones, and higher blood pressure, all of which are linked to hardening of the arteries.

An episode of intense anger doubles the risk of a heart attack within the next two hours. For this reason, stopping to analyze the situation may allow you to realize that anger is an inappropriate and ineffective response and may give you time to choose a less dangerous and more productive reaction.

Sometimes, anger may be the most appropriate response. In such situations, deep breathing, relaxation, and physical activity can defuse and dissipate the anger and help you avoid the negative consequences.

When you feel angry, take 10 slow deep breaths, smile, even if you have to force it, and then respond to the situation.

Positive Passions

Blue Mondays

German researchers analyzed data from nearly 3,000 patients and found that most heart attacks occur on Monday mornings (the least occur on Saturdays). Most of these cardiac events occur during the morning and afternoon hours with the fewest in the wee hours before dawn.

More heart attacks likewise happen in December and January, peaking between Christmas and New Year's Eve. Also, heart attack risk increases during any 24- to 48-hour-period when the temperature drops 18 degrees or more below the average temperature for that day.

Researchers also note that the risk of dying for evening heart attack victims is twice as high as for daytime heart attack victims. Stress reduction, decreased salt intake, and moderation of alcohol intake along with increased physical activity may offer protection during these critical times

Dr. Larry Dossey reminds us that job dissatisfaction is a strong risk factor for a heart attack and that most heart attacks occur on Monday morning at nine o'clock.

Even if you love your job, you need to leave your troubles at work. Those who can leave the rigors of the workplace behind them when they get home have a 67% decreased risk of having a heart attack compared to those who cannot relax and continue fretting over work issues when they get home. Prescribe a little rest and relaxation for yourself and leave your worries at the workplace.

Be Kind to Nurses

Likewise, a four-year study of over 20,000 U.S. nurses found that job stress was a significant factor in their declining physical and mental health, especially for those nurses who felt a lack of control in their jobs, high demands, and low social support. Perhaps we should send flowers to the nurses instead of the patients.

Health Yourself

Stress and Cancer

Researchers from Ohio State University found that reducing stress results in increased levels of tumor-fighting chemicals in women with breast cancer. These more relaxed women were able to tolerate higher doses of chemotherapy, felt less depressed, had more energy, and experienced an overall better quality of life.

High Anxiety: A New Kind of Stress Test

Doctors asked patients with heart disease to give a five-minute speech on an unpleasant topic and scanned their hearts during the speech. Over half the patients had reduced blood flow to the heart as a result of the stress. Those patients who experienced the decreased circulation had three times the risk of death compared to those whose circulation remained normal. Scientists suggest that frequent episodes of stress and anxiety in these patients could prove fatal.

American Heart Association experts say that learning to control anxiety through meditation, exercise, or biofeedback may be as important to heart health as having normal cholesterol levels.

Half Full or Half Empty?

It's also important to avoid the special on going kind of stress caused by pessimism. Defined as a negative outlook on life, pessimism may also be a risk factor for premature death, according to a recent article in the *MBHN*. Mayo Clinic researchers found that pessimists have an increased risk of death, an overall lower level of physical health, a higher risk of depression, and an increased usage of medical resources and higher health care costs.

Research results presented at a prestigious medical conference and published in *Internal Medicine News* show that those having an optimistic outlook on life have better lung function than pessimists. A negative outlook results in a loss of lung function equivalent to smoking a pack a day for 20 years.

Positive Passions

We do not fully understand the connection between positive thinking and health, but researchers think one link is that positive thoughts stimulate hormones that enhance the immune system. Investigators found that people had higher levels of body defenses on days that they described themselves as "feeling good."

But here's the optimistic outlook: Dr. Martin Seligman, author of *Learned Optimism*, found that a group of college students were able to improve their optimism after eight weeks of training and they also experienced an increase in their health status. Start seeing the glass as half full and breathe easier.

Animal House II

Researchers at the American Psychosomatic Society found that couples who own cats or dogs have healthier relationships than couples without pets. Couples with pets responded better to stress, were more satisfied with marriage, and had closer relationships with their spouses.

Researchers measured heart rate and blood pressure levels during stress and found that those couples with pets had lower blood pressure levels before the stress and also got back to normal more quickly than their petless counterparts.

Say It with Flowers

Flowers trigger positive emotions, increase feelings of satisfaction, have a positive effect on behavior, and give us an emotional edge that can last for several days. Scientific studies now show that recipients of flowers experience these benefits. Other than the financial impact, researchers are unsure of the effect on the sender, but common sense and experience tells us it feels pretty good to send flowers, too.

Health Yourself

A Dose of Humor

Commercial airline pilots, those who fly the passenger jets, must pass a rigorous physical examination every six months. I once had a pilot who passed his physical except for a moderately high blood pressure. He'd never had any blood pressure problems before, but I could not certify him until his blood pressure readings were normal. My nurse rechecked his blood pressure several times but it never budged, even when we had him lie down and close his eyes. Finally, I gave him a humorous publication to read and 10 minutes later he was laughing his head off and his blood pressure dropped well below the required level.

This is not a surprise to those of us who are aware of the healing properties of humor and laughter. Dr. Norman Cousins refers to laughter as "intestinal jogging" and notes that laughter and humor lower sensitivity to pain, reduce stress, and improve your body's immune (defense) system.

According to wellness experts Dr. David Sobel and Dr. Robert Ornstein, laughing exercises muscles of the face, shoulder, diaphragm, and abdomen, resulting in elevated heart rates and blood pressure levels as well as increased oxygen in the bloodstream. Laughter acts just like other forms of exercise and burns as many calories per hour as brisk walking. Like exercise, laughter produces lower blood pressure, relaxed muscles, and improved moods afterwards. During laughter your brain produces endorphins – chemicals that reduce the sensation of pain and increase the levels of mental alertness and well-being.

Dr. Sobel, editor of the *MBHN*, says doctors may one day prescribe humorous videos to help patients recover from heart attacks. Dr. Sobel notes that a team of researchers studied a group of heart attack patients, all of whom received standard medical care and an exercise program, but half of them also watched a humorous video of their choice every day. After a year, those who watched the funny videos had lower blood pressures, fewer irregular heartbeats, and lower levels of stress hormones. The humor group also required less medication and only 20% of them had a repeat heart attack, compared to 50% of the usual care group.

Positive Passions

Here are some tips to increase your humor potential and help you prescribe humor and laughter for yourself:

- Add humor to your everyday existence. Read humorous books and stories and watch videos with a humor or comedy theme.
- Put up cartoons in your home and workplace.
- Seek out and hang around people with a healthy sense of humor.
- Write down, remember, and share the funny "little things" that happen each day.
- Laugh at yourself first. We all have plenty of real life experiences we can use to make others laugh.
- Always look for the "funny side" of stressful or negative events in your life. These situations can take on a positive "spin" if you recognize the humor in them.

Dr. Sobel reminds us that people who can laugh at themselves have a much stronger sense of self-worth and higher self-esteem than those who cannot laugh at themselves.

Pass It On

Once when my family was vacationing in the Oregon wilderness, our camper truck's battery died. We were miles from the nearest town and it was a Sunday. I hiked several miles to get to a phone and called a mechanic in the next town 40 miles away. A few hours later Roy, the mechanic, showed up and jump-started our comatose camper. I feared Roy would really soak me financially for providing this service, especially once he found out I was a doctor. When I asked him "How much do I owe you?" Roy replied, "Nothing."

"What? *Nothing*?"

"That's right," Roy said as he pointed to the braces on his paralyzed leg.

"When I was in Vietnam I got shot and a buddy risked his life to save me.

Health Yourself

I asked him how I could ever repay him and he said, 'Just remember me by passing it on to the next poor guy who needs a hand.'" Roy added, "You can pay me back by passing it on whenever you get the chance."

Roy and his rescuer were practicing an activity known as altruism, the act of helping someone out with no expectation of anything in return. Besides being good for our fellow man and benefiting society, unselfish acts of altruism can have a positive impact on your health. Researchers at the University of Michigan surveyed a group of 1,200 retirees and found that over a third regularly donated time to charitable activities or organizations. Those who volunteered lived longer than those who were not involved in giving of their time and efforts. People who gave up to 40 hours a year to a single cause were 40% more likely to be alive at the end of the eight-year study. Those who divided the same amount of time among several different projects did not experience the same advantage.

UCLA psychiatrist Dr. Arnold Schiebel explained the effect: "Being busy, having a sense of commitment – a sense of being something other than passive and useless – is very positive for health."

Look for opportunities to "pass it on" and find ways to assist others with no expectation of gratitude or return on your investment of altruism. Equally important is cultivating the humility to be on the receiving end of beneficent acts. This frame of mind may be more difficult than it sounds. Several years ago when we were forced out of our flood-ravaged home, we found ourselves in temporary quarters in friends' homes, we were fed by the Salvation Army and Red Cross volunteers, and we were the recipients of relief packages from church, school, and civic groups. I was very uncomfortable in this role of "refugee" until I later realized that unless someone is willing to receive help, there can be no opportunity for others to practice the rewarding act of altruism.

Health Yourself Smarter

The explosion of medical information available today from a seemingly

Positive Passions

infinite number of sources makes it difficult for those of us who have a keen interest in health and wellness to evaluate the reliability of the information. This situation is compounded by the fact that the traditional source of medical information, the family doctor, may be increasingly unavailable to help sort through the overabundance of data and information.

Just as you are now deputized to take on more responsibility and be your own "doctor" in some situations, you must now become your own expert in evaluating the medical studies, reports, and articles that you see in the media and on the Internet.

Carol Newman's article, "How to Be a Savvy Health Information Consumer" in *RFN*, offers nine guidelines to help you have confidence in the sources of information you find on medical and health issues:

> 1. "Understand the difference between evidence-based and anecdotal." When you hear that "Uncle Jake smoked like a chimney and outlived his brothers," that's anecdotal. There is no evidence to link smoking to Uncle Jake's longevity.
>
> Evidence-based in this illustrated case means that there are measurable differences between a group that smokes and one that doesn't, and that other factors are taken into consideration.
>
> 2. "Develop healthy skepticism." Just like your parents warned you, if it sounds too good to be true, it probably is. Headlines and claims like "Vitamins Cure Baldness" should be taken with a healthy dose of skepticism.
>
> 3. Always ask yourself, "Who's selling what?" Slick salesmen and entrepreneurs can manipulate information to make it deceptively attractive.
>
> 4. Follow the money. Find out who funded the research. Research paid for by companies who stand to profit from a product's success cannot be considered independent research. Independent research means the study was done by those who are indifferent to the results.
>
> 5. Look for signs of high-quality research. It's easy to tell good bananas from bad ones, but evaluating research is not quite as easy. Positive signs for research include whether or not the study was randomized, meaning that subjects in the study are assigned by chance to one of several groups. "Placebo-controlled" means that there must be at least two groups, including one that does not receive the experimental treatment. "Double-blind" refers to the fact that neither the subjects nor the researchers know which patient is in which group. Studies that have larger numbers of subjects are more reliable than those involving fewer numbers.

6. When you see the phrase "preliminary findings," translate it to mean that the research needs to be repeated and verified before it can yield a recommendation.

7. Human research is often influenced and confused by emotional and psychological factors that cannot always be detected or explained.

8. Don't compare apples to oranges. Animal research findings may not apply to humans.

9. Beware of "one man shows" on the Internet. Web sites of professional organizations, nonprofit agencies, and government agencies may be more reliable.

Conclusion: Keep It All in Perspective

I had just completed giving a presentation on "The Candy, Booze, and Sex Prescription" when an elderly gentleman in the front row raised his hand and spoke.

"Doc, I've added up all the percentages you mentioned and by my calculation I should live forever."

He was joking, of course, but he made a valid point. Making better choices does not confer immortality. If you choose three recommendations that each lowers the risk of heart attack by 50%, it does not mean that your protection from heart attacks triples. My mother made the same mental mistake when she bought her first washing machine. The salesman told her, "This machine will cut your workload in half."

"Good," replied my mother. "I'll take two of them."

The percentages reported in research studies apply only to those who participated in the study. That the research participants experienced a certain level of benefit does not necessarily translate as an equal benefit for the general population. Research results indicate a trend or probability that may hold true for the general public. As mentioned earlier, always discuss any proposed changes in your healthcare practices with your doctor and health care team before implementing new activities or approaches.

Positive Passions

With that said, I challenge each of you to write and fill your own prescription for "Candy, Booze, and Sex" as you practice PRO-vention and health yourself.

About the Author

Dr. Ken Davis is a board-certified family physician with 25 years of practice experience. He received his medical degree from the University of Texas Medical Branch in Galveston, Texas, and completed his specialty training at a UCLA affiliated residency program. Dr. Davis is on the faculty at his alma mater, UTMB, and also at the University of Texas Health Science Center of Houston.

He is an author and professional speaker who addresses national and international audiences on a wide variety of medical and non-medical topics.

Dr. Davis has served as a residency program director, managed care medical director, and has been extensively involved in organized medicine at the local, state, and national levels.

He and his wife Kitty live in Conroe, Texas, and have two grown daughters. His community involvement projects include church activities, charitable fundraising, and volunteer work.

He is an avid baseball fan and enjoys bicycling, running, and racquetball.